Polio: A Dose of the Refiner's Fire

Surviving Polio

by

Jeane L. Curey Dille

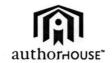

authorHOUSE™

1663 LIBERTY DRIVE, SUITE 200
BLOOMINGTON, INDIANA 47403
(800) 839-8640
WWW.AUTHORHOUSE.COM

First published by AuthorHouse 12/30/04

ISBN: 1-4208-0393-X (sc)

Printed in the United States of America
Bloomington, Indiana

This book is printed on acid-free paper.

Chapter I: It's Not the Flu

In our home, the milkman woke us with his 5 o'clock morning delivery. In the 1950s, milkmen delivered dairy products door-to-door from delivery trucks. Getting up early offered quiet time before I woke my husband, Bill, and the children. Cynthia was five and had just started kindergarten. Linda was a lively, 19-month toddler. My usual routine, after dressing, was to open the front porch door, pick up two glass milk bottles in each hand and take the milk to the refrigerator. But this day, two of the four bottles fell to the floor intact; only glass shards and streaming white liquid remained of the other two bottles. I stared at the mess in disbelief, realizing that my hands and shoulders did not obey my commands.

Weakness, pain and frustration swept over me. I was too weak to stand and my shoulders screamed with pain when I tried to be upright. I spent much time kneeling over the toilet being sick. During these sessions, it was almost impossible to keep my toddler out of the bathroom. Knowing that this was not "just a case of the flu," I tried masking my face, washing my hands often, and keeping distance from the rest of the family to reduce the chance of contagion. These were good intentions, but not always successful. My toddler wanted her usual attentions—the playing, reading and rocking. But the red handkerchief mask frightened her. She still had to be fed, bathed and diapered. There was no one else to do it.

After Bill went to work in the morning and Cynthia left for school, I tried to watch Linda. Most of the time, I laid on the sofa because of severe weakness and because, in a supine position, my shoulders experienced less pain. The only way I could pull myself into a sitting position was by hooking the outside foot around the bottom of the sofa frame. I was afraid to lie on the floor because of extreme weakness and without the use of my arms, I might be unable to get back on my feet again.

Somehow, that day passed. However, the next day going up and down the steep stairs to the bedrooms became impossible. Overall weakness and jarring pain made the steps an insurmountable effort. So, Bill put a mattress on the floor downstairs next to the bathroom for me to sleep on.

In desperation, I called Sandy Day, a teenager who had been my part-time babysitter for a year while I did secretarial work at home. When she understood the situation, with her parents' permission, she offered to stay days with us. She was a mature fourteen-year-old, the eldest child whose mother had taught her well. She realized (as did her parents) that this could be and was a serious illness. Despite knowing the potential danger, her parents gave permission for her to "skip" school to take over the job of daytime housekeeper and nurse.

I believe she stayed a week; maybe it was ten days. Anyhow, she stayed until the hospital had room for me. So far as I have been able to find out, no one caught the illness from me. During that month of October 1952, no one else from the little town of Albion, Michigan was sent to Battle Creek, the designated regional center for polio.

Sandy knew the rhythm of our house. With her there to maintain the routine, the children were less apprehensive. Sandy made the meals, did the laundry, straightened the house, and cared for Linda who was not yet toilet-trained. Also, during the day, Sandy performed the duties of a first-class special nurse. Because I was a bed (or mattress) patient, she bathed, fed, dressed, and offered me the bedpan. At night, Bill took over. Although I don't remember it, he later told me that he administered hot packs at night to assuage the pain in my shoulders and back.

After the incident of the broken milk bottles, I felt pain in the back of my neck that didn't seem related to the flu symptoms of the previous week. Daily the weakness increased. Books, radio, newspapers and television programs featured polio-related information: statistics, theories about contagion, and descriptions of symptoms. The first intuition that what I was experiencing could be polio-related came from earlier reading. Like most parents of young children, I had a consuming need for information about how and where it was transmitted. Only a few weeks before, one television account described a woman with bulbar (respiratory) polio who delivered a full-term infant while in an iron lung. There were to be many similarities between our experiences.

The moment the bottles fell from my hands, "polio" flashed across my mind. After I described the symptoms of weakened hands, back, shoulder, and neck pain to the doctor on the telephone, Dr. Alice Campbell, made a house call. She took special interest in whether my neck would bend, how far it could be bent forward and how far the chin could be bent down. After her first examination, she told me, "I don't find a stiff neck, I find a sore neck. Go to bed and maybe you won't have the rest of the symptoms." Neither one of us spoke the dread word, "polio," but we both understood what was implied.

Two days later, during the doctor's next visit on Friday, she stated she found a stiff neck. In fact, the neck was rigid. My head would turn neither side-to-side nor up-and-down. This rigidity confirmed her diagnosis. Dr. Campbell's diagnosis was officially confirmed later by a spinal tap when I arrived at the hospital. My sensation was not what I normally felt in the neck area between my shoulder blades and up through the back of the head. Now it felt as if that particular area were filled with a rigid, three-inch board.

After Dr. Campbell confirmed her diagnosis about 8 o'clock on that Friday evening, she used our phone to call the hospital. But there was no room at the hospital that night, nor the next day. The hospital in Calhoun County, where we lived, designated for polio victims was Leila-Post Montgomery Hospital in Battle Creek, an hour from where we lived. Word that the hospital could accommodate me Sunday afternoon raised my spirits. I was certain that the doctors would perform miracles—that I would be cured, good as new, and back home in time to take my daughters tricks-and-treating for Halloween was less than two weeks away.

When the ambulance arrived early Sunday afternoon, only the owner of the service appeared. Both his driver and the driver's assistant had refused the assignment. Probably they feared exposure to themselves or that they might bring the sickness to their families. So the owner did the driving and my husband, Bill, assumed the duties of assistant.

The children's grandparents came to pick them up just before the ambulance left. As parents, we were concerned about the health of our children. The grandparents anguished over the welfare of their grandchildren. Neither child had shown any symptoms other than a cold. The day before, the pediatrician had given the children gamma globulin shots. He explained that even though the shots would not prevent the onset of polio, they might improve the children's immune systems.

Knowing I might never see them again, I wanted to hold them in my arms and crush the warmth of their bodies against me one more time and feel the wetness of their kisses. But I mustn't call them to me or touch them. I tried to grin and send them off with a weak, "I love you." Smiling as they turned away, each child took a grandparent by the hand and danced out the door.

Lacking both the energy to change clothes or the desire to incur the pain such movements would involve, what I wore would have to suffice. Over pajamas, I wore a scratchy woolen robe which irritated my skin. Although I was burning with fever, at the same time, I was also shivering with cold. I couldn't raise my arms to comb my shoulder-length hair because of weakness and pain, so neat hair was no longer a priority. Also, anything touching my head hurt. In fact, I felt pain more places than I can describe. I must have looked extremely disheveled because Bill, who never commented on my appearance, offered to brush my hair before we left for the hospital. I agreed. But after a few strokes, I could tolerate no more. Hair would have to remain as it was.

After parking his ambulance in front of the house, the owner brought a stretcher into the front room. With two or three straps, he fastened me to the frame so he and Bill could carry the load down the front steps and ease it into the back of the ambulance. Once inside, the stretcher and I were fastened down with more straps across the chest, midsection, and ankles. I recall thinking, "What a waste to put those restraints on my upper body." I could neither sit up nor raise my arms. In fact, even breathing required effort.

Once in the hospital parking lot, we stopped at a back entrance. The ensuing trip can best be described as "the scenic route." Probably fear surrounding polio and ignorance of how it was spread determined the route. After being transferred to a gurney wagon (a stretcher with wheels), we traveled areas that represented the least exposure, the minimum danger, to other humans. I was rolled, feet-first, down corridors at various levels. Overhead passage lights furnished my landscape. I counted the lights as they flashed by between turns.

Records of my arrival at the hospital show that I was first examined as an outpatient. What I remember of the exam is a quiet, sympathetic doctor who spoke with an accent. He explained that he had to perform a spinal tap for diagnostic purposes. (Six months earlier I had taken my father-in-law for tests which included a spinal tap for other than a polio diagnosis.) According to Dad, the tap was an excruciatingly painful process. But realizing that I didn't have an alternative, I consented to the spinal tap procedure. The young doctor asked me to lie on my side and curl myself into a ball. I complied, or tried to. Again he asked me to curl into a ball. I told him, "I am." Evidently what he saw was a rather straight spine. He smiled and proceeded. He understood that no additional curling was possible. To my relief, all I felt was a slight needle prick. On the same exam record, I see the signature of a kind and understanding man, Dr. Roman. Even though he was not my primary physician, Dr. Roman and I would meet again on several occasions and soon.

Just after noon that Sunday in October, the ambulance had left my home in Albion—the last time I was to see that home. It was late afternoon or early evening. Bill must have departed with the ambulance driver. Anyway, I don't recall seeing him again that day.

How I arrived at my assigned room, who dressed me in a hospital gown and transferred me to bed escapes recall. My first memory is of awakening the following morning long before daylight in a dimly-lit, all-white, hospital room. The only bed, mine, faced the distant door. To my right were some white-painted metal lockers. Next to them, a door opened into a small, utilitarian bath. Windows on the left wall looked across into windows of the parallel wing. At the far end of the room facing me was that far-away door which led to the hall. Beside the door stood a clothes rack—the only piece of furniture other than the bed and my tray table. Everything in the room was white except the metal bed frame. The room gave stark, stripped-for-action, desolate ambience.

Later, after daylight when I again awakened, a nurse wearing a white surgical mask and gown stood by the bed.

She showed me where the "call" button was pinned to the sheet by my left hand (my left, my better side), told me that I was in isolation, and that my doctor, Dr. Lee Shipp, would see me the next morning. Was there anything else I needed? Yes, there was. I had no pillow, could I have one? She answered that it was better for me to lie flat. But I was uncomfortable lying flat. I wanted, felt I needed, must have a pillow. The nurse said she would look into the matter.

For the first time, I watched the routine which would be repeated whenever anyone left or entered this isolation room. The routine followed this sequence: Those leaving washed their hands in the adjoining bath and walked to the clothes rack which stood next to the hallway door. The long-sleeved, white surgical gown and mask were removed and hung on the clothes rack. Only then did they open the hallway door, step into the hall, and close the door behind them with a metallic click. I was alone in this stark-white silent room with questions, loneliness, fear, and desperation chasing each other in my mind. I tried to replace them by fastening on the first meeting with my doctor, assuring myself that by some mysterious means, he would make me well and return me to my home and family.

Somewhat later the nurse returned with the answer to my request for a pillow. The doctor still maintained that lying flat was better than using a standard pillow. However, he had suggested an alternative. She held up a small, four-or-five-inch diameter, doughnut-shaped affair. It was the kind of pillow, she explained, that hemorrhoid patients sat on after surgery. If I could be content with something this size (new, of course), the doctor would agree. I gave it a try. It wasn't what I had in mind or was accustomed to, but it did make me more comfortable.

To cheer myself and to distract my frightening thoughts, I tried to imagine what the great Dr. Shipp would look like. I fantasized that when he arrived on his rounds the next morning, he would perform some miracle which would heal me quickly and completely. Wishful thinking assured me that all doctors were great healers. They were like gods. All I had to do was hang in there through the night, until his visit the following morning. Then, with a wave of the great Dr. Shipp's powerful hand, I would be fully restored to my former strength and powers, immediately discharged, and rejoin my beloved family almost before they had a chance to miss me.

Of his first visit, I remember little except the aura of strength he exuded and his good humor. Soon I discovered that he told at least one joke each day. Further, that these jokes occurred at the point when I posed a question concerning my prognosis. The humor, I realized, served two purposes; it provided a distraction as well as a transition to other subjects. In effect, it forced me to become more practical. I began to accept that I wouldn't be cured with a wave of his hand, a shot, or a dose of medicine. Slowly and reluctantly I realized that neither Dr. Shipp nor anyone else could predict what would happen that day much less in the future.

To be honest, ever since Dr. Campbell had pronounced the word "polio," I had known this siege would be neither short-term nor easy. But I hadn't permitted myself to believe it. Searching my memory for jokes to match those Dr. Shipp had told was but one of the ways I passed the time between his daily visits.

He didn't heal me the first visit or prescribe any magical potion. However, he did recommend the visit of an eye, ear, nose and throat specialist because I was having more problems with fluid drainage. Dr. Shipp had ordered intravenous liquids (IVs) which I mistakenly attributed to the inability to feed myself. (This inability was due to my almost useless arms and flat position.) My assumption was incorrect. My occasional problem with swallowing had been noted. The IVs were to prevent dehydration.

Later that morning, Dr. Carl Wenke, the throat specialist, introduced himself. I recall him as a tall, slender, elderly, white-haired, bespectacled individual who exuded warmth. He looked in my nose, mouth, and throat; chatted briefly about my condition and my family; and left with the casual remark that I should let the nurses know if the drainage increased or if I had problems swallowing.

For the first few days, time seemed elastic. It passed incredibly slowly. The room was so white, so quiet, so empty. Isolation was broken only by the doctors' daily visits and the presence of the nurses when I had to call them. Otherwise, the door remained closed. None of the sounds or activities of the hallway filtered into the room. To fill my mind and to battle against encroaching dark thoughts, I concentrated on the last church service I attended two weeks before. The passage from Psalms 46 kept whirling, like a carousel, in my head. The first three verses:

> "God is our refuge and strength, a very present help in trouble. Therefore, will not we fear, though the earth be removed, and though the mountains be carried into the midst of the sea; Though the waters thereof roar and be troubled; though the mountains shake with the swelling thereof. There is a river, the streams whereof shall make glad the city of God, the holy place of the tabernacles of the Most High. God is in the midst of her; she shall not be moved; God shall help her, and that right early."

I repeated endlessly to myself. But I wanted and needed the following verses. Someone brought a bible so the nurses could read the missing verses to me because I was unable to hold a book.

Often unusual events, utterly unlike hospital routines, confused me. I realized they were hallucinations, but I was powerless to stop them. I awakened in the middle of the night while it was still dark certain that it was already breakfast time. Instead of lying in a bed, I thought I was

9

lying on a brown, leather pad like an extension of a chair. Believing breakfast was ready, I felt impelled to brush my teeth and rinse my mouth. Because my hands didn't respond to my will, I spilled enough water in the bed to make it uncomfortably wet and cold. When the nurse did arrive, she changed the bed and added more covers to make me warm. Long periods of uninterrupted time were hazy from drifting in and out of consciousness.

During daylight, I noticed clouds of dust kept forming and re-forming above me on the ceiling. Interestingly, the clouds assumed identifiable forms—one of which was Arthur Godfrey, a current radio star. Other famous figures cavorted on the ceiling of my room. On the one hand, I noted and identified these individuals. But in my conscious mind, I knew that these images were not real, that the clouds really were not there, and this truly was not a filthy hospital filled with clouds of dust. Later I came to appreciate what a really fine, efficiently-run, well maintained hospital I was fortunate to be in.

Someone brought a radio to keep me company during the endless, worry-filled hours of isolation. A nurse called my attention to a newscaster reporting that an iron lung was being sped under police escort with sirens from Ann Arbor to Battle Creek (where I was). At the time I found this to be of only passing interest. Not until the day I left, three months later, did I discover that particular piece of equipment was intended for me. Covered with sheets, the iron lung remained, a silent reminder, outside the door of my room when I was discharged. It had been provided in case the chest respirator was not sufficient—in the event my breathing difficulties became severe enough to require the lung. Incidentally, at that time the iron lung equipment was called a "Drinker." Possibly the name came from the man who invented it or perhaps from the company which produced it. Anyway, when I left Leila-Post Montgomery Hospital, a Drinker, draped in sheets, still stood guard outside my door.

Tuesday, my second day in the hospital, during one of the many times I don't remember, one of the nurses gave me a bed bath. I knew when I awoke that I had clean, dry linen. Also, I was pleased to discover that she (I am assuming it was a female) had brushed and braided my long, flyaway hair into two braids. No doubt it looked better. My head, which was so sensitive to pressure and pain, rested more easily. That nurse had also positioned me on my left side with one pillow between my knees and another pillow behind me to brace my back. I felt clean, warm, and more comfortable than I had been in weeks. But I can't remember seeing her because I was not conscious of her presence and didn't awaken until after she left. Possibly she saw me as a young wife in isolation, going through the crisis of a form of disease which conferred almost certain death. Her hands conveyed love and concern together with practiced, soothing training. No remembrance of hands, face, or voice accompanied her action. Never was there a chance to thank her because I never discovered who she was.

That same night was the experience nearest to Hell I can imagine. Time after time I surprised myself by herding great numbers of Communists into the small, adjoining bathroom. I was convinced they were there, up to no good, and that someone had to come and take them from me into custodial care. During this time Communists were being hunted as ominous threats to our national security. I suppose these hallucinations may have been triggered by the media-created frenzy. Newspapers and television wallowed in publicizing Senator Joe McCarthy's Senate hearings. The apparent purpose of the hearings was to investigate suspected Communist activities. Certainly, the hearings created some political entities such as Joe McCarthy and Richard Nixon in the process.

Perhaps a few of those questioned and persecuted in the McCarthy sessions were actually guilty. Certainly many were tried and incarcerated as a threat to the nation. However, some, when questioned, were coerced or frightened into naming friends or associates. A great many individuals, although blameless, were stigmatized to the point where they had neither friends nor employment in their own country. Like Paul Robeson, who held national stature as a lawyer, Shakespearean and movie actor, consummate musician, and football player; they were forced to leave the country in order to work and to protect their families. And when Robeson did return in 1976 to make his professional comeback, he was murdered in Philadelphia—the same year we celebrated America's 200th anniversary. The same year that Martin Luther King was murdered.

In my delirium, I had slipped out of bed to capture all those so-called Communist individuals. But once out of bed, I awakened sharply aware of the weight of my arms making my shoulders scream with pain. So I dragged myself back to the bed and draped the useless upper half of my body across the mattress. Unable to get back into bed by myself, I rang the bell and waited for the nurse's assistance. Always it took her a long time to answer my call. And these Communist roundups required my presence several times during the night.

After each roundup, realizing that I was hallucinating, in agony I begged the nurse to put side rails on the bed or to restrain me. She was gracious about helping me back into bed, but she explained that she couldn't arrange for the restraints. She was alone on duty with 36 patients during the night shift. She had no one to send for the equipment until her relief came in the morning. And each time she was called, she repeated The Routine required by isolation rules when entering the room, nor did she forget to reverse them when leaving. Whether it was for emergency or not, I was still in isolation. That meant she had to don mask and gown when she entered; wash and divest herself of the mask and gown when she left. These, I understood, were regulations.

By morning, I no longer needed restraints. The situation had changed drastically.

After Tuesday night's strenuous activities, I awoke terrified to find my chest covered with a rubber-like shell called a respirator or cuirass. Whatever was done to me and who was involved were a complete mystery. The shell, rounded in front over my chest, began as low as the pelvic bones and reached to the base of the neck. The front of the shell was fastened around the back of the upper body with two, broad, suspender-like elastic bands. A flexible tube joined the top of the shell to a motor-driven vacuum machine. During Dr. Shipp's morning visit, he explained what I had quickly understood: the machine's operation took over the breathing muscles' function. He spoke of another patient who had a similar breathing problem. The patient's father, a farmer, had modified a milking machine to assist his son's breathing. With his usual humor, Dr. Shipp tapped on the respirator shell and quipped that it would do miracles for my figure.

Dr. Wencke also visited me early that same day. He repeated his solemn advice that I should alert the nurses if the nasal drainage increased. I thought him prophetic because within a few hours, drainage became profuse and swallowing problems increased. Soon after complaining to the nurse of increasing drainage, Dr. Wencke appeared. We chatted a little while about nothing in particular while he examined my nose and throat (and observed the drainage). Then he asked where my husband, Bill, was at this time and how he could be reached. I thought to myself, "How kind this was of the doctor and how did he know that Wednesday was Bill's afternoon off?" Dr. Wencke also mentioned that the additional drainage was of concern because it could possibly block the airway. This blockage was to be avoided if at all possible in my situation. When one is in a respirator, the machine determines WHEN one inhales and exhales. In addition, it determines HOW OFTEN and HOW DEEPLY one breathes. Both of us knew that I didn't have the necessary muscle strength to cough should I need to clear the airway myself. I could blink my eyes, move my mouth and head, had some little use of the left arm; but the rest of the muscles from neck to waist did not respond.

Although I don't recall seeing Bill before the procedure, he must have been present because I have a copy of the release he signed on that date giving consent to do a surgical procedure—a tracheotomy. Soon a very cheerful Dr. Wencke introduced Dr. Roman, the sympathetic doctor who performed the spinal tap when I arrived at the hospital. He also introduced the Catholic sister who would be his assisting nurse. Again, my earlier reading had alerted me that this "little procedure" we were discussing was probably going to be a tracheotomy. The opening created by the tracheotomy was essential to ensure a clear airway from which phlegm or drainage could be removed by suction. Because I could neither cough nor blow my nose, a tracheotomy was the alternative.

Because this was still during the two-weeks' isolation period, surgery would be performed here in my hospital room. General anesthesia was not an option since it would further depress respiration. Instead, the Nembutol suppository I was given produced an effect similar to twilight sleep. It dulled the edges of the pain, but still I was awake and more or less alert.

Dr. Wencke, the surgical nurse, and the surgical tray were on the left side of my bed. Dr. Roman sat in the chair on my right holding my powerless right hand. I might have been more upset had there not been a cloth over my eyes. Through the entire procedure, Dr. Wencke kept explaining what he was doing and what was happening. Possibly this was an instructional process for Dr. Roman's benefit. Not only was it a learning experience, but it also kept me informed and more accepting about what was happening to me.

My interest in Dr. Wencke's continuing description of the procedure held my attention and kept the time from dragging. At one point, he asked the nurse to hand him something. Evidently she wasn't quick enough or didn't offer the needed item. In exasperation, he dropped or threw something glass on the floor where it shattered. He continued. When he said "Now when you get between the 3rd and 4th (or was it 4th and 5th?) . . ." he made his puncture incision into the cartilage in the front of my neck and inserted the bell-or funnel-shaped device that slipped into the opening. When I felt the impact of the puncture, I tried to raise up. But it was a futile gesture because I was held in place by the respirator and Dr. Roman's reassuring hand. As I think of it now, I marvel that the doctor was able to be so precise. When the respirator caused me to inhale, it also arched my back causing a slight movement of my head toward the respirator. When the machine's vacuum ceased and I exhaled, my head and neck moved back to their former positions, thus making the neck area a constantly-moving target.

Much of what I describe came through sensations my body communicated—Dr. Roman holding my hand, the cloth blindfold over my eyes, the sound of breaking glass, and the pounding on my neck to puncture the incision for the tracheotomy and the cool sensation when Dr. Wencke inserted the tube into my neck. Dr. Wencke's continuing narrative provided more details and understanding.

But on another level, I experienced a more compelling revelation. At the same time my body rested on the hospital bed I was floating near the ceiling looking down on the four of us. I saw myself in the bed with Dr. Roman leaning over me and watching me intently. Dr. Wencke, swathed in surgical whites towered over the shorter, white-robed surgical nurse. Between the two stood the instrument tray. Dr. Wencke's hands moved busily between my neck and the nurse's hands as she offered him requested instruments. I could hear the swish of material when his arms moved from me back along his side toward the nurse. As I observed the panorama below me, I knew that I was at a dividing point. A nameless, all-powerful expected my highest truth. Without pleadings or promises, wordlessly I expressed my single, dearest wish: that I be permitted to raise my two children. Music, money, power, "things," were inconsequential. Only the rearing of my children was important. However, if sufficient lifetime to rear them were not permitted, I would accept that decision as well. No pronouncements were heard, no decisions of which I was aware. No sounds of thunder or flashes of lightning. I merely found myself back in the hospital bed.

All this must have been over in a relatively short time—probably by mid-afternoon. But the next thing I remember was Dr. Wencke coming into the room. I could see through the window darkness had fallen. In fact, it was late evening. He didn't do The Routine! He headed directly for my bed, bent over me, kissed me on the forehead, and said, "I didn't think I would see you again, sweetheart." Against my cheek and neck I felt the snowflakes from his woolen overcoat. Then he told me that he had been to a reading of "Don Juan in Hell" with Vincent Price, whose surname matched my maiden name and whose work I always admired. I made a mental note to read that play. I shall put reading it on my "to do" list.

Visiting hours were still in effect when Dr. Wencke left that evening. I was surprised and pleased to have another visitor, my husband. He looked harried and disheveled. He said he had been in the waiting room during the surgery. Afterward, he was permitted to visit my room but the surgical mess had not yet been cleaned up. Even though Bill was a butcher and meat cutter by trade, accustomed to seeing and working around blood, seeing the bloody residue around me made him ill. In fact, according to the nurse, he had fainted in the waiting room. Obviously he was not very comfortable in the environment because he said little more than greetings and goodbye. But I felt better for his visit even though I couldn't yet talk.

Sister, Dr. Wencke's surgical nurse, stayed with me after surgery until a special nurse came to take over. Although, technically, special nurses are in charge of maintaining the cleanliness and order of the room, at first the special concentrated on watching my breathing with the new tracheotomy tube. They watched for signs that drainage was clogging my throat, nose, or the tracheotomy "bell," the glass tube that opened out like a flower or funnel. When they heard or spied a warning, they flipped on the switch of the aspirator (vacuum) machine situated on the right side bed table and aimed the straw-sized rubber suction tube at nose, mouth or tracheotomy bell— wherever they thought the phlegm was blocking. In this case, congestion was like drowning in one's own discharge or choking on vomit. Even though I was a superlative long-distance swimmer, drowning was not a preferred way to oblivion.

After the surgery, I had special nurses around-the-clock. Nurses were very scarce, but because of the seriousness of the situation (and requiring almost continuous aspiration) nurses had finally been found. After I awoke and the drainage came, it was my responsibility to point with my still usable left first finger to the place where the mucus was: the nose, the mouth, or the tracheotomy tube. Then the nurse used the aspirator to remove the mass and clear the airway. Dr. Wencke's orders to the nurse were, "Stick the suction tube down until she chokes, then you will know you have it." Incidentally, one does not speak with a tracheotomy tube because the air comes and goes through the trache opening; it does not pass the voice box. A day or two later, Dr. Wencke showed me how to put my usable left forefinger over the trache opening when I wanted to speak. Covering the hole permitted air to pass the voice box, making it possible to use my voice.

I dreaded the three shifts when the new "specials" came for the first time to take over my care because the doctor hadn't yet shown me how to use my voice. As each new person arrived, terror made me wonder, "Just how will we communicate? Will she understand which place I need suction." Nurse and I would eye one another and wonder just what the situation would be. A trust level was at stake. But, somehow, we always reached agreement. Before I could speak, communication was a fearsome problem. Finally, one afternoon, the nurse provided me with a metal fork. She told me to bang on the metal bed frame when I needed attention. This I could do with the left hand. And it worked well until I could close the hole with my finger and let the voice work.

The day after surgery I acquired a roommate, Carol. She was a sixteen-year-old country girl who had quit school for a small job. Her weakness was in her legs, from the waist down. Mine was from the waist to my chin. Later we joked about how between us, we could make one good unit. Moving another bed into the room made it a bit crowded. After days of isolation, broken only by brief visits from Bill, I welcomed the company. Even though our beds faced one another, I couldn't see her because the top of the respirator hid her from view. We enjoyed getting acquainted and having someone to talk with.

From the standpoints of efficiency and logistics, one nurse could "special" two patients. However, both of us were dependent in almost every aspect. Most of the routines were performed during the day, so the day special nurse had her hands full.

We were still in isolation so our visitors were limited to immediate family. For my visitors, a round trip to the hospital took over two hours after a day's work and checking on things at home. Although I tried my best to concentrate on minding the doctor and the healing process, my heart was heavy. It was impossible to screen out worries about who would take care of the children and how they were being cared for. Sandy had gone back to school after ten days of caring for me. My stepfather, who was recuperating from hernia surgery, took over for a day or two, but he found that keeping track of a 19-month-old exceeded both strength and lifting limitations. A neighbor, whom the children adored, stayed until she became ill with a gall bladder attack in the middle of the night. She woke Cynthia, our five-year-old, and sent her around the block alone in the dark to ask the neighbor's husband to help. After that, Bill found a foreign family of three with a young baby to move in. Learning that my toddler and their baby were swapping drinks from the same bottle upset me, nor was I pleased that Linda had reverted to the bottle. But there was little I could do about it so I tried to direct my thoughts elsewhere.

My "baby," Linda, was not the outgoing, social, easy-going type. She was strong-willed and serious. At that time there were few people she would come to or be comfortable with: her father, the beloved neighbor, Sandy, and me. On the other hand, her elder sister, Cynthia, seemed to be at home and at ease almost anywhere. I sometimes described Cynthia as part Gypsy because she loved to travel and was so at ease with people. Because she seemed so mature, I often thought she was born a hundred years old. She didn't miss anything and she seemed to understand everything.

In serious moments, when I allowed myself to consider that I might not return to my family, I was concerned about who would take care of my beloved children. So far as my mother and stepfather were concerned, Cynthia could do no wrong and Linda (the left-hander), could do nothing right. Much the opposite was true of Bill's family. Cynthia was more like the city girl their son had married and, for them, the sun shone brightest on Linda who seemed to love life on the farm.

Missing home and children was a continuous heavy weight; it felt like I was carrying a rock in my stomach. Keeping my thoughts fastened on the situation immediately at hand required constant effort. Yet, when I least expected it, my mind wandered back to how things were at home. Were the children well taken care of? Were they frightened? How was their father handling the responsibilities of keeping the home routine and supervising the children in addition to the demands of his work? Of the two children, I was more concerned about Linda, the toddler. She didn't make friends easily. Like many homes where father works and mother stays home, she had spent more time with me and her sister during her waking hours. We three made much of playtime rituals and rough-and-tumble activities. Because of her age, Linda spent most of her time at home. On the other hand, Cynthia went to school, played with friends across the street, often overnighted at her grandparents', and was often invited by her favorite neighbor for lunch.

Reading had been a special evening pastime with Cynthia almost from the time she was born. Linda soon had her favorites from the Childcraft book series. Cynthia had progressed from nursery rhymes into fairy tales and mysteries. Linda especially liked the poem about The Three Little Kittens. She requested frequent repetitions of the part where the mother says, "You naughty kittens, you've lost your mittens." She liked the "You naughty kittens" part and mimicked the tones even though she couldn't pronounce all of the words. In fact, during one of his hospital visits, Bill asked me what those sounds were, what did she want? He said Linda wanted something and she wanted it badly, but nobody could figure out what it was. I knew immediately that she wanted to have her special poem read to her. She particularly wanted to hear the part about "You naughty kittens." And evidently that was what she wanted because Bill reported she seemed satisfied after that poem was read (and repeated countless times).

Finally, after two weeks, isolation was lifted. Now, friends as well as family were permitted, and bless their hearts, they did. And, our room was back on the roster of hospital rooms to be cleaned and maintained. Housekeeping members were apprehensive about cleaning what had been considered a dangerous isolation area. But since isolation was, by rule, over, they no longer had an excuse. Prior to the end of isolation, our evening nurse, Moselle Cotton, got tired of crunching on the glass shards left over from the surgical procedure. She marched out to the boom closet, returned with broom and dustpan, and triumphantly dumped the swept-up residue into the garbage.

Moselle was one of the most beautiful and talented colored women I have been privileged to meet. To my way of thinking, in addition to being an outstanding nurse, she was beautiful both inside and out. Her mother was Parisian French who married Moselle's father during World War I. Believe me, I hesitated before summoning anyone as elegant as Moselle by drumming a fork against the metal bed frame (even though it was she who had thought to give me the fork). Soon we developed a warm and lasting friendship. It was she I could talk with and confide in during her afternoon shift. During evening visiting hours, when company visited, Moselle absented herself. She felt that her absence gave patients and their visitors more privacy. But that doesn't mean Moselle spent the night relaxing. On one occasion, she showed me a gorgeous, blue chiffon nightgown accompanied by a thank-you note and a check to purchase matching slippers. This beautifully-wrapped gift came from a patient who had been admitted with locked bowels (or severe constipation) with orders that she be given enemas to clear the blockage. The regular nurses had not had sufficient time to follow through, so Moselle offered her services. Moselle proudly announced, "I give enemas high and hot." (I soon had proof of that statement.) Because of Moselle's successful enema technique, the lady was able to leave the hospital that very evening at the end of visiting hours. I don't know whether Moselle was more pleased with the card and gift or with the evidence of her success.

For several days after being placed in the respirator and breathing through the surgically-placed tracheotomy tube, IVs provided nourishment. When I complained that I was hungry, Dr. Shipp asked if I thought I could eat food. My answer was, "Just bring it on. I'm hungry!" Nurses had to feed me most of the 1,000 calorie-a-day diet because my hands didn't work very well. Besides, with the respirator shell curved high over my chest, there was no place to put the food where I could reach much less see it. But it was real food! When Moselle first put a tiny dish of raw celery and carrots next to my left hand where I could feel for and reach it, feeding myself even that small amount was a great accomplishment. To everyone's surprise, swallowing was no longer a problem. I was able to eat everything on the diet. In fact, I was so successful that I gained girth if not weight. The elastic bands which held the respirator in place got so tight they chafed the skin. In fact, they rubbed it raw.

After the nurse pointed out the skin irritation and its cause to Dr. Shipp, he ordered a 750 calorie-a-day diet. I accused him of saving on the hospital's food budget. Within a week, as a result of the new diet, the respirator fit better and I was more comfortable. No more sore, red marks where the elastic bands had rubbed against the skin of my sides and back.

Even though the rule on isolation had been lifted, food delivery and serving remained the same, strange system as before. Those who brought food trays to other patients did not enter our room. Our trays were delivered to our special nurse who brought the food from them into the room for us. Carol's headboard could be raised. This made her sit high enough to feed herself. However, my bed had to remain level (on account of the respirator). This meant I still couldn't see the food or feed myself. If it weren't for having the opportunity to chat with the nurse while she fed me, I would have felt even more like a baby being spoon-fed.

We recognized many not-so-subtle differences from the system used to feed other patients. All of our food came on or in disposable containers. Not even the trays came into our room. We could hear the other china, porcelain, and metal food utensils in the hall. Our eating tools were paper plates, paper cups, and paper containers. Metallic eating tools were washed by our nurse in our bathroom and stored there by her for use with the next meal. When we had finished our repasts, nurse disposed of all paper dishes and leftover food materials in the bathroom wastebasket (which was now emptied daily). No doubt the material from our wastebasket was considered contaminated and disposed of in whatever "hazardous waste material" facility available at the time. Although, by regulation, we were no longer considered infectious, that was only a tentative assumption. The hospital was taking minimal risk that our eating equipment might still be contaminated with some of the dreaded polio virus. No one yet knew how the virus was transmitted or how long it incubated. So the hospital was taking all possible precautions.

Even though solid food represented a step closer to normal eating routine (and possibly some progress toward wellness), the fact that breathed-in air did not pass through my nose inhibited my sense of smell and taste. In fact, everything tasted like the cardboard it came in or on. How I looked forward to the morning "hot" coffee, even though it came in a cardboard container, had little coffee taste, and was more tepid than hot. Maybe it didn't taste like coffee, it had a suggestion of warmth. But expectation was soon tempered by the fact that, when lying flat, liquids must be sipped through a bent straw. And to my shock and dismay, anything warm (such as coffee or cooked cereal), felt as though it would return as soon as I swallowed it. Even though the head of my bed of my bed had long been propped up on six-inch blocks (to assist in drainage), this didn't compensate for the difference in gravity inherent in an upright or sitting position.

Eating and drinking with a tracheotomy and a respirator are, at first, scary. During normal respiration, breathing and swallowing are mutually exclusive. That is, one does not breathe while swallowing. Ordinarily, mixing those two actions causes severe coughing spasms. But a respirator and most other breathing devices are mechanically set to: how many breaths per minute, the duration of each inspiration, how deep (pressure) the inspiration, and how long the release of pressure (expiration). Normally, one automatically stops breathing in order to swallow. But how to swallow when the machine doesn't quit? I said to myself: "You asked for food, you said you could eat it, and here it is. Nobody explained how; just go ahead and do it." Still, I wondered, "Shall I swallow at the the top of the breath, when I am fully inflated, or shall I wait until the bottom of the breath when the pressure is released?"

It's not a problem! The first time I tried swallowing, I felt like I was going down the steep hill on the roller coaster. I didn't know what to expect. My mind was made up. I said a prayer and swallowed. Meanwhile, the respirator continued its rhythmic pulse without interruption, the trache tube didn't clog up, and the food stayed down. Swallowing and breathing at the same time is a sensation like no other. In this particular situation, swallowing can be done anytime during the breathing cycle.

Now that Carol and I were both coherent, past the fever stage, considered stable, and shared the service of one special nurse for each of the three shifts, our weekday routines were fairly predictable. Although our special nurses took vital signs several times daily, as required for our charts, Mrs. Beeson (the 7-3 day nurse whom we soon called "Beeson"), had the heaviest assignment during her day shift. She carried out most of the routines. The night shift (11-7) was leaving when the day shift lights were turned on. Just before the shifts changed, the night nurse took our temperatures and brought us warm, wet washcloths for our hands and faces. Soon afterward, Mrs. Beeson arrived, breakfast arrived. She took the food off of the trays, recovered the silver from the bathroom, served our breakfast, and helped us eat it. Again, Carol was more facile with the eating tools than was I. After the paper and plastic had been deposited in the waste, Beeson washed the eating utensils which remained in our room and put them away for use with the next meal. Next in the order of the day came baths.

Since Carol was paralyzed from the waist down and I was respirator-dependent, had all-but-useless arms (and we didn't yet know about the legs); neither of us was permitted or able to tippy-toe over to the bathtub in the room adjoining. Carol was bathed first, possibly because she was less complicated. While the head of her bed was still cranked up from eating breakfast, she could brush her teeth, wash her face and upper torso. After finishing that part of the bath, the head of her bed was lowered. Beeson took over from there, always careful to cover all but the part being washed. (This is standard procedure to protect the patient from catching cold—maybe consideration for modesty, too.)

After Carol's bath was completed and the water disposed of, Beeson made the bed—with Carol in it, of course. First, Beeson removed the soiled linen from one side of the bed and replaced it with clean linen on that one side. She made the remaining half of the clean linen into a horizontal, sausage-shape which she tucked as far as she could underneath Carol. Then Beeson rolled Carol over the sausage onto the clean side and finished by replacing the linen on the second side. After her bath, Carol could manage her own hair and makeup whenever she chose. It was her legs which were totally useless at this point.

After Carol was clean and processed, Beeson started my bath. Although my legs seemed to respond, there was still the problem of almost-useless arms and how to clean under the respirator. Again, Beeson started from the top. But there were interesting stops along the way. This is no reflection on the nurse's technique or training. But even though it was an improvement, having someone else brush my teeth while they were still in my mouth was far from satisfactory. But we made do. It was either that or go without.

Again, the order of the day was to bathe me from one end to the other. In order to accomplish this, to wash my torso, Beeson had to unsnap the respirator straps, take it off of me, and lay it to the side. I panicked. I felt choked, unable to breathe, and terribly frightened. Getting used to the respirator had taken courage, but now it was my security blanket. Without it, I was certain I would die.

During the first bath, Beeson washed my chest and abdomen deliberately but swiftly, then quickly strapped me back into the respirator. All the while I was hungry for air, gasping like a fish out of water. Each succeeding day, she prolonged the time I was outside the respirator. She always watched me carefully, but she made me plead and beg for her to reattach the breathing machine. Sometimes I thought I would gasp my last before she dried me enough to put back the flannel cloth that separated my chest from the respirator. At last, she snapped the straps back into place. No one had mentioned "frog breathing" which permits people to swallow air for short periods of time when they need breathing assistance. Maybe no one knew about frog breathing for humans during the early 50s although I suspect someone did.

But bulbar polio, one of the three strains of that disease, is the strain which affects the breathing apparatus. Research indicates that, of the three polio strains, bulbar polio is most apt to be fatal. On the other hand, statistically, those who do survive it are not so likely to sustain paralysis. At one point during hospitalization, I was told that I was the first adult to survive polio—at least in that geographical area.

Beeson's next routine was to hot pack us. Wrapping polio patients in heated moist woolen cloths (an innovation discovered by the Australian bush nurse, Sister Kenny) was known to reduce the pain of sore muscles. Hot packs also tended to keep the affected muscles more pliable.

To produce steaming hot cloths for wrapping us, a machine appeared. As I recall, it was called by its trade name, "Singer." The device looked like a three-quart, covered, electric pot supported by three legs. About two feet high, of a silver-like metal, it resembled a big cooking pot on a tripod. As soon as Beeson arrived in the morning, she plugged in the Singer so the heating unit would begin producing steam to heat the woolen cloths inside. The cloths, as I recall, were about 24 by 36 inches; the machine could hold four of these. Carol's two legs and my two arms each required a cloth, so the steamer must have held at least four.

Beeson's method of hot-packing was different from others I have encountered. She was taught to expose the affected area, lift the steaming cloth out of the steamer with some sort of grabbing tool, and wave the hot cloth in the air until enough heat was dissipated that the patient could tolerate having the cloth placed on his skin. So far, the routine is standard. The departure from other methods of wrapping came after she wrapped the limb. Instead of stopping there, she covered the cloth with clear plastic and secured the cloth and plastic wrapping with several safety pins. This pack lasted for two hours rather than the usual 20-30 minutes.

By the time Beeson gave us our baths, changed our beds, and gave us our morning hot packs, doctors were making their rounds. During their morning visits, Carol and I were comfy and warm wrapped in our steamy cloths. Dr. Shipp would first chat about our progress. Then he would tell his daily joke and I would try to return one in kind. Dr. Wencke always came by to check my progress before he changed the dressing that held the tracheotomy bell (that funnel-shaped metal piece whose narrow, straw-size tube was inserted in my neck to keep the airway open). Then he cleaned the opening before he secured another, sterile bell in place with narrow adhesive tape.

One day, in Dr. Wencke's absence, his assistant came by, accompanied by half a dozen individuals—perhaps residents or students. With large motions and lengthy eloquence, he removed the narrow tape and bell. After cleaning, when he attached a different, sterile bell, he proudly secured it with wide, two-inch adhesive. Dr. Wencke became noticeably angry the following day as he began to remove the wide tape and replace the bell. Immediately he realized how painful it was to pull all that wide tape from sensitive neck skin. He understood, as well, what an ignorant, grandstand play his assistant had made. We didn't discuss it, although he made sure I knew of his displeasure. His vehement comment was, "That will never happen again!"

Soon after the doctors left, lunch arrived. By this time, the hot packs were at least two hours old. Also, they were stone cold. But lunch with the cold wraps was next. Only after lunch was over would Beeson replace the cold wraps with hot ones. As I look back now, I wonder that we didn't catch pneumonia from being wet and cold. But that wasn't the end of it. Before she left at the end of her shift in mid afternoon, she placed the damp cloths back in the Singer pot where they remained all night. After a couple of weeks of 24-hour wetness, these woolen cloths took on a perfume of their own. As the aroma waxed in strength, our appetites for lunch waned. Soon, Moselle, our afternoon nurse, began sniffing around to find out "what died." There weren't many possibilities. She soon located the source. No, she didn't get new cloths. She just proceeded to wash them out in the tub each afternoon or evening and hang them up somewhere in the bathroom. Beeson never seemed to notice that the clothes no longer reeked. Perhaps her nose didn't pick up the odor. In other matters, Beeson took great pains about being careful, clean, and efficient.

Although Moselle didn't comment directly, she did mention that at one time in Chicago, on her shift, she cared for 14 patients all of whom were in iron lungs. This suggested that there were more efficient ways of caring for bulbar patients if she was able to handle 14 of them, giving each one trache (tracheotomy) care as well as hot packs. On the other hand, it may also have indicated that the ratio of nurses to patients was limited because of the scarcity of nurses, the population of patients involved, or the fear that everyone had in regard to caring for patients.

Now that we were out of isolation, the promised physical therapy could begin. We had been counting the days and hours. Probably Carol was not aware, but I knew that the longer we went without therapy, the greater probability of stiffness and muscle loss. During the week, the therapist came to our room twice a day. She exercised and stretched our arms and legs. Many times we were told, "Use it or lose it!" We heard that and another refrain, "No smart, no cure!" repeated constantly. The exercises, not always pleasant, were necessary to preserve range of motion so the muscles wouldn't shrink, freeze, or atrophy. Our therapist went through range-of-motion with my left arm without much difficulty. But the muscles of the right arm were a different story. Already they had begun to stiffen noticeably and painfully. In addition to the therapist's exercises, in the afternoon Moselle sandbagged my right arm out away from my side. She stretched the arm as far as she could (as far as I could tolerate) and sandbagged it in that position as long as I could stand it. Although I moaned and complained during the process, for this, among other things, I owe her much.

Carol frequently had afternoon visitors. She lived in Battle Creek, the same area as the hospital, so it was not uncommon to see her family and friends. That is, I could see them if they were where the respirator didn't impede my view. For the most part, Carol's outlook remained optimistic. Two boyfriends came to visit her. She had made plans to marry one. But he came at ever greater intervals and finally disappeared. The other one visited regularly, was always interested in her progress, and seemed undaunted with the news that probably she would always have to use crutches and wear full-length leg braces.

But when her fiance began losing interest, visiting less often, she became quiet, listless, and uncooperative. She picked at her food, spoke little and refused visitors at one point. I asked the nurse about a visiting teacher. Surprise! One came by; but Carol was not interested. However, the teacher and I had long talks. Thanks to the pulsing of the respirator motor, Carol could distinguish nothing of what we said. But knowing Carol's speaking pattern, her dislike for school, and her background in farming; I felt she was ill-prepared to achieve her own independence. Not that there is anything wrong with farming, but with crutches and braces, physically she would be unable to resume that lifestyle. And the prognosis for Carol was permanent paralysis and full-length leg braces augmented by crutches.

So when we had time to ourselves, Carol and I talked about a lot of things, including our future. I suggested some possibilities, some of which interested her enough that she wanted to find out more about them. Finally, she expressed interest in the home teacher. Between Carol and the teacher, they worked in the direction of her interests. I was able to follow Carol's progress on a limited basis after Christmas when we were both discharged from the hospital. But she did return to school and she did marry the steady beau, not the earlier fiance.

After the two weeks' isolation, the physical therapist and the orthopedist were able to accomplish a great deal with Carol still in our room. The therapist came twice a day on weekdays. She did range-of-motion exercises to keep the leg muscles supple and some elementary exercises of the upper extremities. The orthopedist recommended shoes with metal sole plates that were to be placed flat against the foot board of the bed. As I understood it, this was to hold the feet in such a position that the hamstrings in the back of her legs would not shorten. Such shortening would lead to a dropped toe and other problems. Although the treatment with shoes and foot board sounded uncomfortable, Carol didn't complain. So it must have been tolerable.

But every staff member who visited insisted that the best therapy for my situation would be water therapy. And that could not be accomplished until and unless I was free of the respirator for at least 24 hours. Essentially, until I could again breathe on my own, there would be no visit to the therapy pool and area. Until my record showed that I could be free of the breathing machine for a 24-hour period, I would have to remain attached to the respirator, inside the room. As a further incentive, after I had been out of the respirator a week or ten days, the trache could be removed.

These were the two goals I fought for with all my strength, endurance, and determination: getting out of the respirator and getting rid of the trache tube. Now I began to appreciate why Beeson dawdled more every day with my bath. She wasn't trying to make me uncomfortable, she was helping me lengthen the time I could breathe unassisted.

With Beeson's help and a lot of encouragement from everyone I talked with, the intervals outside the machine steadily lengthened. In fact, they both lengthened and became more frequent during the day. By Thanksgiving week, I could breathe half a day on my own although I was unable to relinquish the machine at night and deeply frightened that I would forget to breathe when I fell asleep. Now, finally, I could see Carol when we talked.

Thanksgiving was the first full day I was able to breathe without the machine. I was ecstatic with my progress, but night time was another matter. The fear of forgetting to breathe in my sleep never left because breathing didn't seem instinctive; it required determined effort. Several times when I drifted off, I was awakened by the metallic click of the locker next to my bed, followed by the crinkling of paper. Nurse Moselle was in my locker dipping into the gifts of candy as I had invited her to do. It was disturbing even though I had made the offer. Had the machine been pumping away, I wouldn't have been able to hear her. But the noise distracted my entry into slumber.

Usually about the middle of the night, I was awakened. This was another part of the regular routine. Carol wasn't yet able to void by herself, so when the pressure became too severe, nurse had to catherize her. That pressure point usually occurred about 2 in the morning. Our night nurse, whose name I cannot remember because I so seldom talked with her, was very short. I do recall that she walked with a limp and wore her hair plaited in braids around her head. She couldn't have been five feet tall because, from my vantage point, she scarcely seemed taller than the bed. I'm sure she was trained and that she knew how to do the catherization procedure, but she just wasn't able to do it because she was so short. So she had to ask the night charge nurse (the same one who had been alone with 35 patients) to interrupt her duties and perform the catherization which would bring Carol relief. The procedure involved a lot of whispering, rustling, and occasional banging of the metal bedpan. After that was over, I steeled myself to go back to sleep. When Beeson came the following morning, I hadn't had to ask for the respirator. I had successfully completed the 24-hour period. Now I waited impatiently to go to physical therapy.

Although the news of my readiness was delivered, this was the Friday after Thanksgiving, part of the Thanksgiving holiday for many staff members. When she started her afternoon shift, no call had come from therapy and it was already 3:00 p.m. Moselle found me in tears. As soon as Moselle discovered the reason for my misery, she hurried out of the room. When she returned a few minutes later, she said she had had to use the phone. (Our room didn't have a phone—most hospital rooms had no phones at that time, so she must have used the one at the nurses' station.)

Shortly after, a young woman with a slight limp wheeled a chair into the room. The therapist who helped Moselle transfer me into the chair didn't look older than sixteen. Making the transfer from the bed to the chair might have been dangerous because I hadn't been on my feet for six weeks. So they took no chances on my ability to stand. As soon as I sat upright, my shoulders were savaged from the weight of my arms until the nurse placed a pillow on my lap to support the weight. Then off we went to the physical therapy department in the bowels of the hospital.

As I was told later, only one therapist was left on duty after the holiday—and her shift had officially ended. She was just leaving when nurse telephoned. Unfortunately, the therapist made the mistake of answering the telephone. She got an earful of vehement language. As a result of the verbal drubbing, she changed her mind about leaving early. In fact, she evidently grabbed a wheelchair at once and hurried to my room.

What I saw of therapy then was a clean but unadorned, cement, shallow pool filled with warm water. The therapist removed the blanket wrapped around me, my slippers, and my hospital gown. She helped me to my feet, pointed toward the pool and told me to go in. (Nobody told me I couldn't walk, so I walked!) I managed the short distance to the edge of the pool, stepped in, and sat down in water up to my chin. My shoulders were quiet; the buoyancy of the water supported my arms. For ten or fifteen minutes, I wiggled everything I could wiggle, which felt marvelous. Then I began to wonder, "How do I get out of here without hands or arms? It's simple. Get up on your knees, stand up, and walk to the edge without stumbling." This I did. At the edge, the therapist met me with a towel, dried me off, and dressed me in gown and slippers. She sat me in the wheelchair, tucked the blanket around me, propped up my arms with the pillow, and wheeled me back to my room. Even after so short a session, I was tired. But I had started real therapy! That was the beginning of regaining whatever muscle strength and use I would be permitted to have.

Even before this, some use of my left arm was returning. Not to the point where I could raise it to wash my face or brush my teeth. But I found out that, while lying down, I was able to hold a paperback book. That was wonderful. Books transported me out of my present environment, blotted out homesickness, erased worries about the family, and made the time pass far more pleasantly. Beeson rose to the occasion. She had a teenage son who loved Westerns. She brought them up by the dozen. Westerns are low priority on my reading list, but I read them two or three a day. The nurse/sister who visited regularly nicknamed me, "Professor" because, she said, I was always reading. After a while I told her the Westerns made me saddle sore, my eyes ached from the dust, and I was tired of all the blood and corpses. But still I read.

During her visits, sister and I had many interesting discussions. Sometimes the topics surprised me because they ranged from marriage to careers to child-rearing. She offered many valuable insights on rearing children based on observations of her sister's family. Probably she knew that these were matters which concerned me. Talking about them gave me a chance to voice some of my concerns. And that helped. She was an interesting person, warm and perceptive. Had it not been for her visits, there were many days I would have had no visitor other than the hospital staff.

After I had been hospitalized nearly a month, I asked Beeson what the date was. In fifteen years my menstrual cycle had been nearly as regular as clockwork. In my mind, there was no doubt about it. I was more than two weeks late. (Now there is evidence that pregnant women are particularly susceptible to polio, but no one knew that then.) Beeson,

Moselle, and I held a great discussion centering on how high fever could throw the body's clock off. Of course, the nurses alerted Dr. Shipp. Without mentioning it to me, Dr. Shipp ordered a pregnancy test. At that time, rabbits were the standard laboratory animal on which pregnancy tests were performed. Dr. Shipp had to be absent the day the results came in. So he told the nurse on duty to let me know the test was negative (that I was not pregnant), but that it was inconclusive because not enough fluid was injected into the rabbit to make the test valid. What he didn't tell the nurse was that he was running another test. So the next time I saw Dr. Shipp, he had the report of the second test. And this time, the test was positive and valid. I was definitely pregnant. When Dr. Shipp asked me if I knew about the rabbit, I answered, "Oh yes, something happened to the rabbit." He later told me he didn't have the heart to tell me right then about the newer positive results. He waited until his next visit to explain the mix-up, the results of the second test, and that I was indeed pregnant.

In the meantime information had filtered all over the hospital floor about that poor, paralyzed woman who had yet to find out she was pregnant. One floor nurse, who was French and who had trained in France, came to visit me. Lots of other staff members came to visit too—probably from kindness, pity, maybe curiosity? But the charming French nurse really distracted and amused me with her little stories. Most of the RNs wore their caps as well as their nursing pins. Each nursing school had its own cap design and one could identify where the nurse had trained by the design of her cap. But this young lady said she didn't wear her cap because it was such an atrocious design. Her declaration piqued my interest, so she promised to bring the hat and model it for me. This she did a few days later. I was still in the respirator and, until she stood on the seat of a chair at my bedside, I couldn't see her. After I saw her wearing the hat, I understood her reluctance to show it. The hat resembled an 18-inch pizza pan. In shape, it resembled a UFO. The halo, itself, was made of white, stiffly-starched, organdy-like material. The fabric was pleated to lie flat like the pizza pan. The little band holding the larger, pan-shaped structure to her head was similar to the landing or cockpit area of the UFO. Laundering and ironing it must have taken hours. No wonder she preferred not to wear it to work. Showing it to me was a warm act of friendship and concern, one I've remembered for more than fifty years.

This happened while I was still in the respirator. It was she, I recall, who whispered to me that other patients on the floor were complaining about the whooshing noise the respirator made. She and the other nurses described my condition and the necessity for the whooshing noise. This put an end to the complaints.

Knowing my concern about the pregnancy, Dr. Shipp sent Dr. Roman and his wife, Dr. Sophie, to see me. These two doctors were Polish refugees who preferred to be called by their given names because people had trouble pronouncing their surname. Dr. Roman had been the first one to check me into the hospital in the Outpatient Department. Also, he was the kindly soul who held my hand and lent his energy and support during the trache operation. He and Dr. Sophie had come to assuage my concerns about pregnancy and to give me encouragement. After Dr. Roman left the room, Dr. Sophie removed the respirator to examine me. After a minute and prolonged examination, she gave her opinion that my breasts were those of a pregnant woman.

Finally, the truth began to seep through my barricade of denial. During Dr. Shipp's visit the next morning, he said he had contacted our family doctor in Jackson about my polio and the associated pregnancy. Dr. Jason Meads had also delivered both of my children. He offered to drive the 50 miles to visit me and check me out. It was a wonderful offer and I appreciated it. But whether I was brash or determined, I declined the offer and said I would wait until I was home.

Then I would go see Dr. Meads. At the time I wouldn't consider that I might not get home. The fact that neither of my children had evidenced signs of polio encouraged me to be upbeat and optimistic.

On the bright side, once I was free of the respirator, I was allowed to be up in a wheelchair twice a day for fifteen minutes. Always a pillow supported my arms. With two pillows on the seat of wheelchair, thirty minutes was more than I could tolerate. Even though the posterior area had suffered no identifiable damage, sitting even for a short time was uncomfortable. Many months would pass before I could sit an hour even with the pillows. After a few days of 2 fifteen-minute sittings, the wheelchair period was extended to half an hour accompanied by permission to meet Bill, my evening visitor, in the lounge. What a treat to meet my visitor outside our hospital room. A real change of venue.

The lounge or visitors' area, so welcome because it offered change from our room, hallways, or physical therapy; tended to be cooler than our room was kept. This was during extremely cold winter weather. The halls were subject to drafts, too. After so much hot-pack therapy, possibly we were intolerant of the cold. Since both Carol and I were considered fairly stable, our private nurses were no longer necessary. In the evening an aide was assigned to change me from nothing but a hospital gown into lounging pajamas because I still could not use my arms to dress myself. The aide was a young, good-looking man in his mid-twenties. At first, I was embarrassed and reluctant to be dressed by this stranger. As he slipped the pajama trousers over my nakedness, he said, "This is just like putting snow pants on my little boy." Bless his heart, that put me more at ease.

Years afterward, my Mother told me she had visited while I was still in isolation. She was not permitted in the room, but she could see me dimly through the window of the parallel wing. She said she cried when she saw me in the respirator. And when she saw how difficult it was when the nurse used the aspirator to clear my airway, she prayed that if I couldn't get better, let me die. When she heard about my pregnancy, she got busy with her sewing machine. (Maybe it is an inherited trait that when someone in our family is concerned about an individual, we sew, cook, write, or knit something for that person.) Mother created two eye-catching lounging pajama outfits. One pajama top had bright stripes trimmed with plain forest green to match the forest green trousers. This outfit I called my Coat of Many Colors. The jacket of the second outfit had pastel flowers with sky-blue trimming which matched the blue pants. When these were brought to me, I really couldn't see them well because the respirator was in the way. The little French nurse offered to model one for me. She tried on the blue-flowered top and stood on a chair seat so I could see what it looked like. I was delighted with the jacket but, at the same time, I have to admit that I was a little jealous that she could wear it (and I couldn't, maybe never would). She was so charming about it, I offered her some of the candy that was accumulating in my locker.

Once formal physical therapy started, a more suitable method of getting me into the pool was inaugurated. After dressing me in a hospital-created muslin bikini-like outfit, I was eased into the pool of warm water. After weeks in bed, the water seemed to caress and massage the length of my body. Aching muscles were soothed; the body was exercised enough to encourage sleep. After my "dip," I don't remember getting out of the pool, but I do remember being transferred from the wheelchair back into the bed with my hair dripping wet.

Rubber bed sheets protected the mattress from the dampness of the hot packs as well as from the moisture from my hair after pool therapy. But after a few weeks of the woolen packs and wet hair, it seemed to me that I smelled like a billy goat. Finally, after a great deal of pleading, I persuaded Moselle to cut my hair short with her bandage scissors. Then she took pity on me and used a dry shampoo which at least removed some of the oil, soil, and aroma. In fact, she used what was then called Minipoo shampoo a couple of times during the eight or nine weeks she was our special nurse.

Toward the end of my stay, another young woman who had been hospitalized with polio came to visit me. She was still an inpatient, but was ambulatory. Maybe it was because I was looking forward to going home for Christmas or perhaps because I was pregnant and depressed, she offered to give me a real, water shampoo while I was in bed. It had to be done in bed because I was not yet mobile. Already we had discovered that I could stand (much to everyone's surprise), but only long enough to transfer to a wheelchair.

Prior to this, Dr. Shipp refused to consider any request for a wet shampoo. But now, to my delight, he gave his permission. My visitor commandeered the shampoo tray and all the rest of the necessary items. Gathering the essentials, alone, took a lot of effort. Then she had to get water and dump the used, soapy water into the bathroom sink. All of this must have demanded a great deal of energy from her. My deepest thanks and a box of candy could not begin to communicate my appreciation. Before, no amount of perfume or talcum could have erased the aroma of perspiration and sour, woolen cloths that followed me; now, after the daily bed bath, I felt clean and had the assurance that my fragrance did not precede me. This act lifted my spirits and raised my self-assurance.

By the time I was able to forego the use of the respirator, the drainage problem had diminished to the point where Dr. Wencke decided it was time to remove the trache tube. He didn't wish to sew the incision in my neck closed. He explained that by leaving the wound to heal by itself, it would be easier and quicker to reinsert the tube should that be necessary. I was glad to be rid of the tube. More significantly, the absence of the tube carried with it the assumption that the aspiration process was a thing of the past. With the trache opening healed over, there would be less chance of infection. Of everything that happened during this hospitalization, the most fearful at the time was the tracheotomy operation. And in retrospect, the most painful was the choking that required aspirating to remove drainage. No wonder I was jubilant to be free of the respirator AND the tube.

In connection with the respirator, two interesting adventures occurred. After I had been on the respirator a few days (round-the-clock, of course), I complained to Moselle that the machine was slowing down. Either my breathing was failing, or else the machine-set sequence was slowing, she assured me that nothing was happening, that my imagination was overactive. At the same time, she kept a steady conversation going, never moving more than a couple of feet from my bedside. In spite of her diverting stories, I began to tense and worry. I was about to cry out in desperation when a maintenance man wheeled in another respirator which he and Moselle quickly activated. Within a minute or two, the second unit was programmed and I was transferred into it, safe and sound. Afterward we concentrated on the timely arrival of the back-up machine. What was not discussed was, what would have happened if the first machine had quit before the second one arrived. CPR was not a highly-touted alternative at that time and conventional lifesaving breathing techniques probably would not have been successful. We waved a fond good-bye to the ailing machine and settled down into our more-or-less comfortable routine.

A few days later, we did a rerun of that adventure. Why it happened again on the afternoon shift is not important. But this time Moselle admitted that the machine was malfunctioning and that the charge nurse had called for a back-up. I wasn't quite as upset by the waiting as I was the previous time, partly because we had gotten through it before and partly because she had leveled with me and I knew what was going on. (However, no one had yet told me about the Drinker, the iron lung, parked outside my door.)

Very soon I discovered why this latest respirator was not their No. 1 or No. 2 unit. Each time the pump produced its vacuum, it made a sound like ka-BOOM, or a pile-driver. At the sound of the BOOM, the respirator shell thumped down on the bony areas which supported it. A thin layer of cloth separated the respirator from my clavicle and pelvic bones. Even though the thumps were not sharp blows, they did have a definite impact—not enough to make bruises or black-and blue marks. But the impact was sufficient to interfere with the nightly getting-to-sleep process. On the other hand, the noise and discomfort caused by the machine strengthened my resolve to get out of the respirator as soon as possible.

Not until the day I left did I understand why Moselle was not more upset about the malfunction of the respirators. She knew that the Drinker sat outside my door ready to be fired up. Perhaps everyone assumed I knew of its presence. Certainly nobody mentioned it. Maybe it was because the respirator was more comfortable and more easy to be weaned from. The iron lung was a far more restrictive environment. Anyhow, I guess everybody else knew that a truly formidable back-up machine was stationed and ready just outside my door. But they still preferred that I use the chest respirator if at all possible.

Meanwhile, up and down the hall, patients were complaining about the noise of the respirators. Each machine had a different tone or voice. All three had a "whoosh-whoosh," but the last one with the Ka-BOOM they found exceptionally annoying. But when patients understood why the machines sang out, they were supportive.

Once we were permitted visitors, Carol frequently had people drop in both afternoon and evening hours. Once she decided to pursue education, the visiting teacher arrived almost daily. Her visits provided a welcome addition to our regular routine. My family home in Albion was an hour distant. Prior to my illness, Bill had been working an evening as well as his regular day job. Even though he gave up the second job, he couldn't visit every day because he had the house and housekeeper to see to as well as the children.

My father lived still further away, in Detroit. He was able to visit only once almost at the end of my hospitalization. In addition to holding a full-time job, he had the full responsibility of caring for my stepmother who was dying of cancer. At least three or four times a week, he would call the hospital in the evening. Moselle talked with him from the phone in the nurses' station. With my stepmother's care and his concern for me (his only child), usually he had taken some libation before he phoned for a progress report. Whenever he was at loss for words and stressed to the max, he would go through the manual of arms accompanying himself by whistling the associated bugle call. This was a holdover from his service in the World War I navy. And, more recently, he was a member of a precision drill team, the Zouaves of Jackson.

Moselle conveyed progress reports to him and related his messages to me. She would prefix his messages with, "I just talked with your dad— boat whistles and all . . . " (which was part of his manual-of-arms routine. Boat whistles and all told me he loved me, cared about me, and wanted to give me the strength of his support—and also that he had fortified himself with a few sips from the bottle.)

Dad's employer arranged for someone to stay with my stepmother so dad could take the train to Battle Creek to see me. Bless his heart. With all his other worries and expenses, he brought me a gift—a watch, the "sweetheart model." As I look back now, I realize that he gave a watch to someone he loved who was under siege or facing death. He gave my mother a watch the night before she was go undergo major surgery for thyroid. When I was fifteen, just prior to my parents' divorce, he gave me a watch (which disappeared a few years later). When he knew my stepmother was dying of cancer, he gave her a watch and new luggage. And on this occasion he realized that, although I was out of the respirator and progressing well, impaired breathing capacity offered a dim future. Even though I didn't realize the significance of it then, I cherished that watch as much as any gift I have ever received.

Soon after the isolation period had ended but while I was still in the breathing machine, our minister's wife surprised me with a visit and a gift of earrings. They were little white flowers. Nurse Beeson put them on me and held a mirror so I could see my reflection. Wearing them made me feel very dressed up. After all, other than a flannel square over my chest separating me from the respirator, they were my sole apparel. We had a wonderful visit. I wore the earrings on several occasions during visiting hour. Moselle and I used to joke that the patient, wearing only lipstick and earrings, entertained visitors. Of course, we simply ignored the flannel and the bedclothes that covered the lower extremities.

Fall shifted gears bringing Michigan heavy winter weather. As the outside temperatures fell, the hospital thermostats maintained their daytime comfort level. But the boilers feeding the radiators operated at reduced levels after evening visiting hours. The umbilical cord connecting the vacuum machine respirator and the high hump of the respirator itself prevented covers from being drawn higher than my waist. Daytime temperatures were within the comfort zone. But when the temperatures dropped, my upper body chilled. I often called upon the night nurse to cover my shoulders with a bath towel or to tuck the bath blanket around my neck. Probably she welcomed the request because lights in our room were dimmed so we could sleep. But she sat quietly in her chair, always nearby and on hand should we need her. Carol's need for catherization and my request for covers were her main concern until it was time for her to go off duty at 7:00 a.m.

Although I was unable to take my daughter, Cynthia, tricks-or-treating, the flip side was that by Thanksgiving, I was out of the respirator. Not only could I SEE my food, I could feed myself. Maybe that is an overstatement.

Born right-handed, eating with the left was more than an act of bravado and chance. But the excitement left me dizzy enough to think I could write, which I really wanted to do. Of course, even with all this progress, I was still lying flat in bed. No matter what position the nurse placed the writing pad in, I could neither write nor print legibly. What I did do was work up a fine case of frustration, close to tears. Moselle calmed me by pointing out that writing was not essential to my health. Further, I should concentrate on the many positive aspects. I shouldn't fret about my younger daughter drinking out of the same baby bottle as the immigrant housekeeper's child. Rather, I should be grateful that both of my children were well, showed no signs of polio, and were reportedly in good spirits.

After Thanksgiving, the nearby downtown buildings were decorated with Christmas lights and decorations. Within our hospital room, we could hear Christmas carols on the radio. For the first time, I heard Mel Torme singing his composition Have Yourself a Merry, Merry Christmas which starts with, "Chestnuts roasting on an open fire . . . ." Now that I was off the respirator, the supporting blocks had been removed from the head of my bed. Now, the head of my bed could be raised a little so I could look out the window. After dark, when the merchants turned on their festive light displays, nurse moved my bed and turned Carol's bed so we could watch the displays. Beyond the other hospital wing we could see the lighted Christmas tree on the top of one of the taller buildings. To this day, whenever I hear Mel Torme's rending of his famous carol, I remember watching the Christmas tree while we listened to his music.

Being in the hospital for several weeks had not dimmed my anticipation of Dr. Shipp's morning visits. I had finally come to accept that he was human, neither God nor magician; his humor was more satisfying than medicine. One morning he brought a lady patient with him on his rounds. He said he had her in the hospital every six months or so because she could tell fortunes for his patients. And his patients thoroughly enjoyed this, as did I. At the time I wondered if this were a frivolous use of hospitalization. Now I realize that the woman had a serious condition for which she had to be hospitalized at intervals. She may have looked healthy and certainly she was mobile; but nevertheless, she was unwell. But how much joy she left us patients with the interesting (positive) fortunes she told.

With the advent of the Christmas season and its attendant rituals and memories, I became more homesick and depressed. I hadn't seen my children since October. When Dr. Shipp visited the next morning, I told him that if he didn't let me see my children, somehow "I was going to break out of this joint." He told his joke, said some soothing words, and went on his way leaving me without an answer. But the next morning, he told me, "If you give me a nice Christmas present, I'll let you go home for Christmas." At first I thought it was a joke. Then I realized it was a promise! His final words were that I had to have a double-armsling jacket before he would let me leave.

It didn't take me long to pass my family the word. Mother and her trusty sewing machine rose to the occasion. From the pattern she used for my lounging pajamas, she made a sleeveless jacket or vest out of heavy muslin. With this garment she enclosed two, yard-long strips of fabric and a dozen, large safety pins. These strips, when pinned at the proper height, supported my all-but-useless arms.

On the day of my departure from the hospital, the sun shone so brightly on the snow and ice that I was all but blinded. The air was cold, crisp, and crystal clear. Among those who came to wish we well was the little French nurse who came to say, "Adieu." Another nurse, Mrs. Green, came in to tell me "Goodbye" and wish me good luck. I didn't remember ever seeing her before and told her so. She didn't seem upset when she answered, "I am the one who put you in the respirator." That was the night I was rounding up Communists in my bathroom. We had a good laugh over that.

Finally, I was dressed in my Coat-of-Many-Colors lounging pajama outfit over which I wore the vest-jacket. The slings were adjusted to support my arms and pinned in place. For the first time in months, I had real shoes and stockings on my feet. When I stood up beside my bed ready for the transfer to the wheelchair, the weight of the shoes made me feel as if my feet were nailed to the floor. My heavy, winter coat was draped around my shoulders and buttoned up the front. There must have been a scarf over my head, I don't remember. Even though it was bitter cold outside, once in the car I felt like a queen with one pillow under me and two pillows supporting my arms. The day I had been hoping and praying for had arrived. Finally, I would see and hold my two precious daughters. At last I was on my way home.

But "home" was not where I had left it. At the time I left Albion in the ambulance, I had looked around the living room with a strange premonition. At the time I wondered if I would ever see it again. Now the home I was going to was not the familiar one. During my time in hospital, Bill received the transfer he had requested. His new assignment was in Jackson, some twenty miles from Albion where we had lived before I was hospitalized. Jackson is the city where, twelve years earlier, I had graduated from high school. And I had worked there for the telephone company before either Bill or I had gone into the service. Although I had been gone from the city for several years, I had spent about ten years of my life there. It was where Bill and I had met and fallen in love. As I left the Battle Creek hospital, I was reminded that Jackson was in Jackson County; further, that Jackson was the polio headquarters for that county which was now my home. If (and when) I needed additional polio-related services, Foote Hospital in Jackson was the place I was assigned to go.

Long before departing for home and again during the trip, I reminded myself of the often-repeated resolve that, once I was on my feet and out of the hospital, I would NEVER return. As I soon discovered, "never" often elicits a negative result.

Until he could find living quarters for five of us in Jackson (which included the Dr. Shipp-ordered-full-time housekeeper), Bill had commuted to work from Albion. On December 17, 1952, I was discharged from the hospital. In the previous week, Bill had performed a major miracle. Not only had he rented most of a house for us to live in, but he had also moved children and furniture, found and hired a housekeeper—all of this in addition to working his full-time job. The housekeeper must have been a miracle worker, too. All was clean, neat, and attractive. Probably most people would have judged our belongings as ranging from mediocre to shabby; but to me, they looked positively elegant. Most of all, the children were there—a little reserved in their new surroundings. Probably more reserved about their strange-appearing mother, but so beautiful and so dear. After a moment's hesitation, they came running to be kissed and hugged. What a magical moment! And what a revelation.

My recent hospitalization, only nine weeks long, had stretched into eternity. The imminent meeting with the children stole my appetite. Bright sunlight and deep cold dominated that winter midafternoon when we arrived. After the first moments of elation, hugs of greeting were shrouded in fog and penetrated with pain after the ride home. Both girls wanted to "own" me. Only then did I begin to realize how terribly sensitive I was to touch. They were so excited, they didn't want to be reminded it was nap time. Finally, when they were tucked away, I gave in to exhaustion and went to bed. So much for "never."

Describing Catherine, our new housekeeper, is like describing my grandmother. White hair framed a rosy face whose mouth and snapping eyes smiled good-naturedly. Her ample, full-bosomed figure and ready energy belied her sixty-odd years. In the past few days, she had skillfully made order out of the chaos of what was probably an "Okie move." A friend from Oklahoma used the term and defined it as "a move where all the furniture is piled helter-skelter on an open pickup truck and moved, without cover, to its destination." However, nothing seemed the worse for wear and I had the good sense not to look too closely or ask for details. Many possessions never surfaced again. To me, it was enough that I was home. This was the homecoming I had dreamed about but feared would never happen.

Farewells from the Battle Creek hospital repeated Dr. Shipp's urgent order to see my own doctor in Jackson about my pregnancy, now about three months along. Dr. Meads had already seen me through two successful pregnancies. Also, he had been our family doctor and my trusted friend for almost fifteen years. Dutifully, I made the appointment to see him the following Monday morning.

When I walked into his office, Dr. Meads took off my coat. I was wearing it cape-like—not to be stylish but because I had both arms in slings and, besides, tightened muscles wouldn't permit themselves to be stuck into the sleeves. When he saw this, tears came to his eyes. I don't believe he would mind if I repeated what he said, "I can think of a lot of people I would rather see like this than you." Our previous visits had been devoted mostly to sharing anecdotes. In the eighth month of a previous pregnancy, I had told him, "I don't think you are worried about me at all." His immediate reply was, "You're right. I'm not." But that was earlier on when I was still the athlete. While in high school, I had asked the family doctor to put me on a diet because I was too heavy. His reply was, "You'd just make a better halfback than girl." A swimmer who can swim five miles has big shoulders, big muscles, and a deep chest.

That was back "when." Now, I was in a different situation. According to the calendar and the rabbit test results included in my hospital record, I was about three months pregnant. And I was no longer Jeanie the athlete. I had been one sick cookie who hadn't yet recovered the use of arms, shoulders, or full breathing. The truth was, no one could tell if, when, or how much use or strength would return. At this point, performing the activities of daily life for myself, by myself, was impossible. Bathing, brushing teeth, dressing myself all required assistance. In addition, I couldn't care for the two children I already had or maintain my home without assistance. What would I do with a new baby? How could I manage? Who could help me? Would anyone help me?

After I sat down across the desk from him, like the good listener he was, Dr. Meads didn't interrupt these unanswerable questions I had been battling with for the past weeks. When I had finished, he put his hand over mine, pressed it gently, looked me in the eye and solemnly said, "It will be all right." Although he asked a few questions while we chatted briefly, he didn't examine me physically.

As my doctor, he urged me to consult an orthopedist immediately to initiate physical therapy. He recommended two ortho specialists in town: Dr. Stolberg and Dr. Deming. In his opinion, they were equally qualified. When I asked for further background about them, he commented that one, Dr. Stolberg, was more talkative and less formal than the other. Dr. Stolberg was my choice because I prefer to be kept informed about what is happening with my body. Right then, Dr. Meads made the appointment for me to visit Dr. Stolberg's office in a few days. As it turned out, I was to meet Carl Stolberg sooner than the appointment. I would meet him in the polio clinic at the hospital in four days.

That Dr. Meads didn't suggest an appointment for our next meeting seemed strange, but there was always the telephone. He reached for my coat, draped it over my shoulders, and dismissed me with the deliberate statement, "Whenever you want to go to the hospital, just call me."

After I left his office, stores in their holiday garb beckoned me. Christmas was less than a week away. In addition to the usual festivities, Christmas Day was also Linda's second birthday. For none of these events had I been able to make preparations. But I was much too tired for shopping—too tired for anything. My only alternative was to return home to the same impossible situation. The grayness of fatigue and shoulder pain closed around me, stronger than the desire for food. Noontime and evening, as soon as the children had eaten, all three of us went to our sleeping places. Willingly I escaped into sleep.

Of the time between visiting Dr. Meads' office and Christmas Eve I have little recollection, even though a significant event occurred. During those few days, my pregnancy terminated painlessly. And I sent a heartfelt prayer of thanks to a benevolent Creator.

Christmas Eve stands out as a very special time, one I remember every Yuletide these forty-odd years since. It was unique because, for a long time, I didn't know whether I would live to see it. And if I did, would I be united with my family? Early Christmas Eve, the outside temperature was fairly mild. A few snowflakes meandered lazily. When we answered a knock at the door, I saw special friends from high school days accompanied by twenty or so young people. With a Merry Christmas greeting, my dearest school friend handed me a gift—a round, homemade, chocolate cake. It was my favorite: chocolate cake inside and chocolate frosting outside. For more than a half hour, the group sang Christmas carols as we stood on the porch. Someone put a shawl around my shoulders. Ever since the rabbit test I had prayed, "Lord, if it be Thy will, let this cup pass from me." As I listened to the carols, I felt the snowflakes fall softly against my face, like a benediction.

I awoke the next morning with a strange thought. On Christmas Day 1950, two years ago to my great delight, Linda was born. This Christmas Day of 1952 I had been relieved of a pregnancy for which I was physically and mentally unprepared. Truly, the loss was through no act of mine. At the same time, I was deeply thankful for the resolution of the problem.

Like the other eight days I had been home, Christmas Day the children frequently stopped their activities to check on me. They vied for attention to reassure themselves I was indeed present. They returned to their own pursuits only to come back in a short while to make yet another verification. Somehow, while the children slept, Catherine procured and decorated a tree. The floor at the base of the tree offered up presents to delight everyone. By the time the wrappings had been removed and the contents inspected or played with, the rug looked like a demolition derby had taken place. Both children were tired and cranky after the excitement wore off. But most of all, I was bone tired. Every part of my body ached. I felt as if I could never move again and every part of me cried out for rest, relief, and quiet.

"Never" came to haunt me again. Dr. Meads' parting words echoed in my ears, "Whenever you want to go to the hospital, just call me." At 4:00 p.m. on that Christmas afternoon, I telephoned him at home. Without preamble, I begged to return to the hospital as soon as possible. He showed neither surprise nor irritation at receiving a call on Christmas Day. I had the feeling he had been expecting it. He assured me that he would call back soon. And call me back he did—in 20 minutes—saying I could enter Foote Hospital the next morning. That I would wish with such fervor and desperation to return to hospital was a shock. Another "never" that boomeranged.

Admittance to Foote Hospital was a comparatively pleasant experience. Being able to enter under my own steam (although weakly) and on my own two feet had a lot to do with the pleasure. Also, this was early morning after a good night's sleep and I was not yet worn out. Dr. Meads had left orders for admitting me, so I was directed to sit in the nearby wheelchair and pushed to my room.

This was a two-bed room with a bath (but no phone), located on the ground floor in the critical care section. Accident victims, patients with heart problems, and others like me who had special needs were residents of that wing. At first I didn't fully appreciate being located at the far end of the wing. Later I came to understand the special privileges our location conferred. We were permitted to read far into the night, long past other patients' "lights out" time. Also, we were allowed to have our husbands visit after visiting hours were officially over. But at first, I had the room by myself.

That first day, one of my lengthy naps was interrupted by a team of maintenance men. They had bolted a pipe so it ran parallel to the mattress but raised two or three feet above the mattress. From this pipe they fastened a trapeze so it hung where I could reach up with my left hand to grasp it. No, it wasn't for a circus act. It was to help me lift myself out of and back into the bed, necessary because my arms couldn't push me up or pull me back in. Although I had been given bathroom privileges, until this time someone had to assist me getting in and out of bed. Using the trapeze with my left arm to raise my hips, I could make the transfer. What a sense of freedom! What power! Even though I didn't have the energy to walk outside the door, no one had to tell me that bathroom privileges didn't include wandering up and down the hospital corridors. In fact, at first, the only way I got outside the room was by being rolled to physical therapy on a gurney wagon. And since physical therapy was located near the emergency and outpatient areas, whenever I was propelled through those areas, aides made certain I wore a surgical mask. The mask was to protect me from any respiratory ailments, colds, or diseases I might be exposed to in the halls.

Miss Holton, head of the Physical Therapy Department, visited me my second day in the hospital. She told me that when she visited me the first day, she found me asleep and I looked as if I needed the sleep more than a visit. Later I found out that Miss Holton, the physical therapist, was the sister of the Miss Holton who had been the Dean of Women at Jackson High School from which had graduated in 1941. During high school, the Dean and I had many meetings. Some concerned the deleterious effects my tumultuous home life had on my academic efforts; some meetings were about scheduling classes around my employment, not to omit a couple of conferences regarding truancy. But the Misses Holton are two of the most respected professional woman I have known.

Miss Holton of the Physical Therapy Department arranged for the special equipment on my bed—the equipment which afforded me the exhilarating sense of independence about getting in and out of bed. Soon I discovered that she was made of far stronger mettle than my former therapist.

The differences between these two women far outweighed their similarities. The therapist at Leila-Post was probably in her twenties. She told me that she had also had polio, that polio accounted for her limp and walking with a dropped toe. She did perform range-of-motion exercises during and after the time I was in the respirator, but she never wanted to cause any pain. Although the "no pain, no gain approach" is not necessarily more effective, usually pain accompanies stretching a muscle. And she backed off at the first sign of pain. Also, when she took me down the first day for water therapy, she stripped me to the buff and directed me—not helped me—into the water. I was strictly on my own. I don't know what would have happened had I fallen. At that time, with little strength and without arms to push, I'm not sure I could have gotten back on my feet. Furthermore, nobody was even sure I could walk. So she was quite a risk-taker with my body.

On the other hand, in addition to her physical therapy training, Miss Holton had been at Warm Springs, Georgia when President Roosevelt was there. Also, she had been in the military. At one point, she told me she had had radiation sickness twice (she didn't indicate any particulars and one simply didn't ask). Once, when her right hand and arm didn't offer enough resistance, she mentioned she was lucky to have been born ambidextrous. She simply switched to the other hand. Miss Holton was what we in the Navy would call "very GI." Her presence dominated the area. When Miss Holton had that grim look, one could hear a pin drop in the department. Everything was done "toot sweet" and strictly according to regulations.

With the Doctors Stolberg and Deming's approval (they shared an office and were really a team), Miss Holton initiated a six-day-a-week routine that included hot packs twice a day for twenty minutes across the shoulders and down the spine to my heels. Morning and midafternoon, two attractive, young, colored ladies brought the Singer steam machine to my room and hot-packed me in bed. They were quick, efficient, and charming. They whipped those woolen cloths out of the machine, flipped them in the air like one flips a bed sheet until enough heat dissipated that my skin didn't feel burnt. Then they laid the bed blanket over the cloths to hold the warmth for about twenty minutes. As they waited for the cloths to cool, they mentioned working with other polio patients. This was the first I had heard other patients in this hospital were being treated for polio.

I remember Irene, one of the girls who gave hot packs. All the children in the polio weekly clinic called her, "Ring." So we called her Ring, too.

In addition to the twice-a-day hot packs six days a week, Ring and her cohort rolled me onto a gurney wagon and pushed me to that part of the therapy area where the Hubbard tank was located. To me, the tank looked like a standard horse-watering tank over which hovered a Budget hoist. While I was still lying on the gurney, I was dressed in a two-piece, muslin bathing suit and then lifted onto a Streicher frame placed on top of another gurney. (This Streicher frame device has a metal-tubing frame covered with canvas. It resembles an Army cot without legs.) The frame was hooked to chains linked to a Budget hoist. Then the frame and I were lifted off of the supporting gurney and deposited in the bubbling water of the tank. After I was in the water, the hooks were removed from one side of the frame so it could be slid out from under me, leaving me floating unsupported in the 102 degree water. Miss Holton tested to make sure the water temperature was 102 degrees.

After twenty minutes or so, a therapist slid the Streicher frame back under me, reattached the hooks, and engaged the Budget hoist to lift me out of the water and back onto the gurney. There I was dried off enough to be dressed in hospital gown and bathrobe, ready to return to my room. Back in the room, I was rolled off the wagon and deposited (still with wet hair) on the bed.

The routine varied one day a week: Wednesday. That morning, Doctors Deming and Stolberg held "clinic." The doctors wanted to see all the polio patients to check their progress. After all of us had been dunked in the tank, we were dressed in dry, hospital-made exercise outfits. We waited on gurneys or in wheelchairs in various areas of the Therapy Department for our turn to be examined. Two young children, a girl and her brother, ages four and six, waited side-by-side in wheelchairs. Only twice did I see them. Joey, a likable, talkative, two-year-old, wore leg braces which looked too heavy for him to manage. Often, while awaiting clinic, he was laid at the opposite end of my gurney facing me after being in the tank. We kept each other company. Joey's father had been stricken by polio the same time as Joey.

Although I never saw him at clinic or met the man, I heard that Joey's father was critical. He died shortly afterwards.

Joey (or probably anyone in leg braces) walked more normally with dry clothing. His diapers were changed two or three times while he waited on my gurney for the doctors to see him. Ring teased him and asked him who wet his pants. Joey answered, "Jeane did." He knew my name and had the sense of humor to tease me. Because of emergencies, one day I wet Joey's pants three times before the doctors saw him and had him walk for them. Afterwards, I was often teased about wetting Joey's pants.

My first meeting with Doctors Stolberg and Deming was at my first therapy clinic in hospital, not the appointment in their office made for me by Dr. Meads. The two men came alongside where I was lying on the gurney. They had read the written report of muscle strength and range, so they knew I had upper appendage and respiratory problems. With a smile, Dr. Stolberg said, "We're going to make a singer out of you." (At least half of singing is respiratory control.) My feisty reply was, "I already AM a singer!" And this had been true. I had studied voice over a ten-year period and had been a church soloist much of that time. But whether I would have the privilege of singing or the strength to do so again remained in the hands of a higher power.

A background of being a church-singer musician provided immediate recall of some of the most beautiful literature. During the long hours in the respirator, when there was nothing to break the monotony of the pulsing machine and the surrounding grey-white walls, I rehearsed in my mind all the song lyrics and all the biblical texts I knew, always returning to "God is my refuge and strength." Even though everything else might seem to go wrong, this thought always renewed my hope and confidence. As a child I had enjoyed listening to my father, mother, and grandfather recite their favorite poetry. When I heard something I liked, I sought it out and memorized it. To pass the time away, I played this poetry over in my mind.

How lucky I was to have available this private library which I could "read" at will. At first, the word pictures and the language caught my imagination. Now I came to appreciate what the poet, Longfellow, meant when he wrote:

"So read from the treasured volume
the poem of thy choice.
And lend to the rhyme of the poet
the beauty of thy voice.
And the night shall be filled with music
And the cares that beset the day
Shall fold their tents like the Arabs
And as silently steal away."

These are the good mind games that released me from the bondage of the present and made tolerable the passing of time. They also provided company so I was not alone during the long, solitary hours. As I read to myself from the library in my mind, the poet spoke to me. He was my company.

While I remained in hospital, those mind games and the hospital routine were The Reality. Home, husband, and children were another world. Certainly it was a form of make-believe; but keeping the two realities separate permitted me to deal with getting through the obstacles of the present. For a while, it seemed as if I were in Disney World and that Disney World was the only reality. Everything outside the hospital was another world. To dwell on the impossible, on being where I could not be or doing things I was unable to do, would have been frustrating, depressing, and counterproductive.

Back in Physical Therapy, Miss Holton could be warm and sympathetic, but she ran a tight ship. Several times she ordered me to do something in "the voice which must be obeyed." Before I was able to say I couldn't do it, or I hesitated because it was painful, she had already flipped me or put me through the motion. She vehemently corrected my, "I can't do it." Her instructions were, "Always express yourself in the positive. Don't use 'I can't;' say, 'I am unable to.'"

She shared other bits of wisdom with me. One that was immediately useful and another that sequestered itself in my mind for the length of time it took me to build the strength to face it. The first was extremely practical and immediately useful: "When you get out of the bathtub (and most bathrooms had only tubs then), place a wet washcloth on the side of the tub. You can grab onto that and it won't slip." The other suggestion came rather off hand, as if she were philosophizing. In essence, she commented that women were more likely to stay married to handicapped husbands than the other way around. Because I didn't have a handicapped husband, the sense of this eluded me for some time.

One Saturday morning session with Miss Holton stands out above all others. I was standing in front of a cupboard in the rehabilitation unit where one learns to manipulate the gizmos of daily living such as doors, steps, handles, knobs, clothing, et. Miss Holton commanded me to reach up over my head and open the cupboard door. Before I remembered I hadn't been able to reach over my head, I reacted. My left arm obeyed the mind's directive; my fingers curled around the cupboard door hardware and I opened the door. For the first time, I knew I was able to reach, not just to the top of my head, but over my head! Miss Holton and I looked at one another in amazement. I found tears dripping off my face and she turned her head away while she wiped her eyes. At this point we both knew that, at least with one arm, I could reach up and above my head.

Here was the realization of at least some of my hopes. The endless hot packs, massages, and stretching were worth all the pain, discomfort, and frustration. Now I could be more independent because I had full range of motion with the left arm and shoulder. That should not be confused with full strength. What it meant was, at least one time (hopefully more than once), I could complete the motion.

The body knows what it can do before the mind is aware. She demanded and, without conscious thought, my body responded. This ability was good news for several reasons. Had I been unable to reach overhead with one arm or the other, the doctors were considering surgery to set one arm so the elbow was perpendicular to the body. Stabilizing the elbow in such a position would permit raising the lower part of the arm and hand upright—over my head. Now there was no further need to consider such surgery!

As of that memorable Saturday, reaching overhead was not only possible, it was real. This is a day I will always remember and cherish. I felt like a cross between the King of the Hill and the Grandest Tiger in the Jungle. Because I was definitely and unchangeably right-handed, I would have preferred the use of the right upper extremity. But given the alternatives—left arm or neither one—I was delighted and deeply grateful for the return I had received.

I had had the two-bed hospital room to myself for only a couple of days when I was introduced to Eleanor Lewis who would be my roommate for several weeks. Mine was the bed near the door; hers was the one by the window. Eleanor was about my age and each of us had two children. Hers were a girl and a boy; mine were two girls. The doctors attributed Eleanor's horrible headaches to a spinal injury or abnormality.

As mother and sister helped Eleanor carry her belongings into the room, she asked whether I minded if she smoked. My answer was an emphatic, "Yes." After her startled reaction, I explained that I had limited breathing capacity. When someone smoked even as far away as the doorway, I felt as if I were choking. This she understood. So she smoked either in the lounge or in the room of other patients who smoked.

In order to treat the spine, the following day Eleanor was placed in a plaster body cast which reached from just under armpits to mid-derriere. The cast controlled the curve of the spine. For the first two days, until the plaster dried completely, she was somewhat uncomfortable. After that, she adjusted to the situation and complained little. Occasionally she mentioned an itch where she couldn't reach to scratch, but for the most part, she tolerated the cast very well. Soon we were close friends. By the time her cast had dried, we both had bathroom privileges, but we stayed in our room.

By my fourth day in Foote Hospital, I was very uncomfortable, twitching and wiggling. Eleanor noticed this and asked what was the matter. After all, with my trapeze equipment, I could swing in and out of bed at will, use the bathroom instead of the bedpan, and even feed myself after a fashion. I should have been content and at ease. But because I was embarrassed, I used slang to answer her. "I think I've got galloping dandruff."

Eleanor wanted to know what that meant. "I think I have 'crabs' or body lice. I'm not sure. I've never had them. But I have this itching in the pubic area. And I can't bend enough to see what it is and I can't even scratch it very well." We agreed it was best to consult a nurse.

The day charge nurse was the one to check with because this took place during the day shift. Even though our room did not have a telephone, it did have two-way communication with the chart room. However, we had discovered, from listening to the aides, that when the daytime charge nurse was not otherwise engaged, she listened in to what was happening in the patients' rooms. Probably eavesdropping on the patients was not a bad idea because then she knew where her nurses and aides were and what they were doing. But, from what else we heard, she was also known to be a blatant gossip. With that in mind, the day nurse was not the ideal person to consult about an intimate problem.

On the other hand, Mrs. Gray, the afternoon charge nurse, was one whose ear was not connected to the mouth. She had a sense of humor that made her easy to talk with.

We decided to wait until that lady came on duty. When Mrs. Gray came by on her afternoon rounds, I mentioned that I had a personal and private problem I'd like to discuss. At once she closed the door behind her and pulled the chair up by my bed.

"OK. What's to discuss?"

My muttered response was, "I think I have crabs.

Immediately she became the efficient nurse, "What makes you think so?"

"Because I itch in the pubic area, but I can't bend my back enough to look and I can't even scratch," I answered, almost in tears.

With a laugh, Mrs. Gray said, "Let's take a look." She pulled the covers down and my hospital gown up so she could inspect the area. "I don't even know what I'm looking for. I've never seen them."

"If crabs are what I've got, there will be little nit eggs, little dark things, stuck to the base of the pubic hair follicles. I've never had them or seen them, but I've read about them."

"Well, I guess that's what I'm seeing," as she leaned down to peer more closely. "But I guess you don't want this to get around, do you? Shall I call your doctor?" With that, she replaced my gown and the bed covers.

Mrs. Gray returned in an hour or so with a big grin on her face. She reported, "I called Dr. Stolberg and told him about your problem. He said, 'Hell, if she'd had a broken leg, I'd have known how to treat her. Better call Jason (Dr. Meads). He'll know what to do.' So I called Jason and he'll drop in when he makes evening rounds."

Dr. Meads appeared later that evening with an ear-to-ear grin. His eyes twinkled as he asked, "How are WE ALL today?"

I was tempted to shout an angry reply, but decided against it. So I answered meekly, "All of us are doing fine, thank you.

But how do we get rid of those critters? Is someone going to have to shave me? Just what IS going to happen?"

As he leaned against the side of the bed, he took my hand. His voice was gentle as he explained that he would direct someone, other than the one we wanted to avoid, to do the treatment. To my great relief, no shaving was involved. The nurse would wash the area with warm water and soap, dry it, and apply mineral oil twice a day for three days. That should take care of the parasites. They would suffocate from the oil. But, in the meantime, I was to use the bedpan, not the toilet. Until the treatment was completed, my using the toilet might infect someone else with the vermin.

Jason (Dr. Meads) was as good as his word. When a nurse came in, she closed the door AND put a screen around my bed (the rooms didn't have curtain dividers, either). A screen meant, "Stay out," just as it does today. But Mrs. Reed and the aides were mystified why I had to have the bedpan and why a nurse had to do some special treatment when I had been able to use the toilet until this time. Nobody came right out and asked the question, but the atmosphere cleared once I was able to resume my own toileting.

At least three of us wondered just where I had picked up these little parasites: Eleanor, Dr. Meads, and I. After spending roughly two months in a hospital, I had spent only nine days at home. Then, only three days in this hospital before the onset of this embarrassing situation. Bill finally admitted that he had picked up "something" and it must have come from the toilet seat at the store where he worked.

A friend, who had nursed polio patients from the 1930s through the 1950s, commented on how attitudes had changed in the intervening years. Having body parasites at that time was considered the equivalent of having a venereal disease. Venereal disease, like menstruation, masturbation, and discussion of "private parts" was a taboo subject. To have an infestation of parasites or the infection of venereal disease brought with it the ultimate embarrassment.

Now, forty-odd years later, I am freely recording it. A few years ago, the slogan about venereal disease was: "it's not a sin to have it, but it is a sin to keep it." Now the attitude seems to be more tolerant. Perhaps that tolerance is due, in part, because drugs have been developed to cure the more common venereal diseases. But, at the time, I was terribly embarrassed to have the problem. And I desperately wanted to keep the information from spreading all through the hospital community.

Those times I was on my feet I wore the double armsling jacket mother had made as a condition for my discharge at Christmas. Wearing it helped avoid strain on the shoulder and arm muscles and, this in turn, reduced the pain. However, the weight was then distributed to the neck muscles and these, in turn, soon hurt because they were also weak. The doctors explained how fortunate I was to be past adolescence. As an adult, the cartilage supporting bones and joints is more mature and less elastic. Had I been a youngster, I probably would have had one or both shoulders hanging at the elbow level.

The doctors also predicted that to achieve maximum muscle tone and strength would require five years. That didn't mean I would be as good as new. It meant that I might look toward improvement for as long as five years. Maybe I would hit the maximum return in less time; but after five years, it was doubtful that any additional improvement could be achieved.

Thanks to Miss Holton's experience and contacts, I was fitted with a vehicle that made me more comfortable. An additional plus was that I was able to do more for myself. The body of this vehicle, at least the main structure, was an old-fashioned, high-backed wicker wheelchair. Miss Holton had a mechanic who volunteered to create solutions. (His son had died not long before of polio.) To the wheelchair, he affixed metal rods which extended up the back panel of the wheelchair beyond my head on either side. At a point about eight inches above my head, these rods were bent at a 90-degree angle so they pointed straight ahead. From the side, they looked like horizontal antenna facing front. About 18 inches from the bend in the rod, leather armslings were connected to brake springs and then to the rods. When I sat in the wheelchair, my elbows were suspended with armslings at chest level from the overhead rods.

But this was only half of the miracle. In addition, this creative mechanic fastened metal brackets to the wheelchair armrests so a lap board could be slipped into the metal brackets. With this arrangement, my arms hovered over a lap tray table. In this position it was easier to eat, wash, brush hair and teeth, read. In general, I was as comfortable as I could be outside of bed and the Hubbard tank. True, I wasn't good at propelling the device. But in addition to being more comfortable, I was also able to accomplish more of the activities of daily life. Previous to this marvelously-adapted wheelchair, I was dependent upon someone else to perform most of these activities for me. As I became more independent, my outlook and disposition improved. I was never able to thank the mechanic, but many times I asked Miss Holton to express my appreciation. If that gentlemen should ever read this and recognize himself, please accept my heartfelt appreciation.

One incident marred the total success of this marvelous vehicle. Nurses and aides became accustomed to placing my food tray on the lap tray. Aides deposited our trays, took the metal covers off the heated dishes and left Eleanor and me to eat by ourselves. On this particular Sunday, the charge nurse was short-handed (and short-tempered). She delivered the tray but placed it on the outer edge of the lap board. The lap board flipped out of its brackets, the tray fell on the floor, dishes shattered, and I was in tears. First of all, I was disappointed because Sunday dinners were always special. Second, I was hungry. Third, because I knew the nurse was short-handed, I really didn't want to call her back. Finally, an aide returned from her dinner to retrieve our trays. She discovered the accident and found an unused tray on the trolley in the hall left over from a patient who had already been discharged. Although the replacement food was barely warm, I did get to eat Sunday dinner

An unusual sequence of events produced the most spectacular Sunday evening of my five-month stay. Ever since I was admitted, orders were that I was to stay away from respiratory infections (RIs). When my beloved roommate, Eleanor, caught a cold, I was transferred to another room. My new roommate was bedridden with a bad back, but her hearing was intact. She overheard male patients in the next room. One of the men had a deep, rumbling laugh which so enchanted her she asked me, the mobile one, to go find out "who dat man wit da laugh be." At her behest, I discovered that the laugh belonged to one who had had back surgery. His roommate, a traveling salesman from out of town, had collided with a semi in the dark before dawn as he was returning from visiting his girlfriend. The salesman's injuries were painful and serious. Among other problems, he had a broken clavicle and some broken ribs. His bed was propped up, but breathing was still painful. And to laugh really hurt! But his roommate laughed joyously and often. And the two of them spent their time trying to top the other's stories.

I conveyed my roommate's curiosity about who was it laughing. Immediately they invited me in. But when I saw they smoked, I parked my wheelchair just outside their doorway so we could talk (and I could breathe). They asked me to invite my roommate, but the present one was unable to walk. So I passed by my former room and asked Eleanor if she wanted to visit since she was mobile. When Eleanor joined us, there were the three smokers in the room and I could still chime in from my position at the doorway.

While we visited, we discovered that the salesman had many acquaintances: lodge brothers, customers, and friends. Most of them brought gifts of beverages. Later we saw that his locker was filled with bottles of liquor. We also learned that the salesman's wife came to visit during afternoons and his girlfriend came evenings.

He asked, "Do you like garlic bread?" We gave an enthusiastic affirmative. He continued, "My girlfriend is coming early this evening and I've asked her to bring some garlic bread. Why don't you come back and join us?" That sounded good to us.

As it turned out, the wife stayed late and the girlfriend came early. So Eleanor and I chatted with the girlfriend in the hall until the wife left. Then we joined the two gentlemen who wondered about ice and soda pop to go with their beverages. I had one of the aides wheel me to the chart room where there was ice and then to the pop machines for bottles of Coke (I was now permitted to go anywhere in the hospital except where there was an RI). Although Eleanor was recovering from her RI, she could take the proffered chair inside the men patients' room. I remained just outside their door to avoid the heavy smoke and the RI. I could see and hear everything as well as enjoy iced Coke, garlic bread, cheese, and some wonderful jokes. The others mixed what they wished and finished the bread. When dinner came, none of us was hungry. The aides were only a little mystified when they took away our trays (and perhaps they ate whatever looked good because we hadn't touched the food).

Between the armsling jacket and my "rocket" wheelchair, I became quite mobile. One of our favorite nurses, "Mrs. Contessa," remained as day charge nurse. Perhaps because of Eleanor's previous hospital stays, associated with her long-standing headache problem, she used more familiar terms of address. So far as Eleanor was concerned, the charge nurse was "Tessie." This familiar address was used in our room, in the chart room, and in the halls. I'm not sure how Eleanor addressed this pleasant and capable nurse in front of doctors or other professionals. It never occurred to me to use this familiar address. Mrs. Contessa gave me permission to go anywhere in the hospital provided: (1) I told someone in the chart room where I was going and, (2) I avoided anybody or any area with an RI.

Dr. Lewis (not our doctor but Eleanor's husband's uncle), visited us almost daily. Eleanor addressed him as "Doc" to which he responded with a warm grin. To me, of course, he was "Dr.Lewis." As soon as Eleanor's cast was set and dried to everyone's satisfaction, she was mobile. She was directed to "walk bent slightly forward with the angle of the cast and swing your arms like a gorilla." On the street she might have been embarrassed, but within the family of our hospital environment, her walk elicited first a hidden smirk and then an outright laugh from staff and newcomers alike. And all of us could use a good laugh.

Although in the back of my mind I realized that my illness had racked up a huge debt in medical bills, that was part of the separate reality I didn't permit myself to dwell on. Worries about home life, children, debts, and future physical ability were kept behind a screen. Perhaps I thought our Blue Cross Insurance underwrote everything illness-related. When Moselle, the evening nurse from my previous hospitalization, visited I made a great discovery. Yes, she had made the fifty-mile trip to visit. But she also needed my husband's signature so she could get her final paycheck for special nursing.

It was then I learned that all my expenses, both in Battle Creek and in Jackson, had been and were being underwritten by the March of Dimes. That organization had covered the costs of hospitalization, special nurses, surgeries, mechanical ventilation, physical therapy to name a few. And the March of Dimes would continue to underwrite my physical therapy, rehabilitation, and yet another surgery over a period of some three years. I was overwhelmed with this knowledge. Even though I had tried to barricade financial worries away from my thoughts, they lurked there in the background waiting to be solved. The solution was awe-inspiring. How much I owed and still owe to this marvelous organization.

After my multiple entities (body lice) had been duly eliminated and I was once again my singular self with permission to use the toilet, Dr. Meads continued to visit daily. He arrived most mornings about an hour before lunch. After inquiring about my condition and offering the joke of the day, he wandered over to the window sill to inspect whatever flowers were there. The buttonhole in the lapel of his suit jacket contained a minute glass flower vase. If the flowers were small and fresh enough, he broke one off and tucked it into the lapel vase fastened to the suit jacket lapel. I recall the single fresh flower and the daily joke as his trademarks.

On the same window sill with the flowers were boxes of whatever "goodies" we had received. These ranged from candy, caramel corn, and cookies, to the equally-welcome mail, books, magazines, and stationery. Dr. Meads inspected the edibles with care and helped himself. Usually when his mouth was full of candy or cookies, he droned on about how he was dieting. This performance was almost as funny as his jokes.

Whenever he was in the building, he stopped at least to say, "Hello." One morning about 5, he came into the room, tugged at my toe and said, "There's been a sleet storm and I won't get to see you this morning. Bye." And he went on about his County Coroner's duties.

Of the professional men who visited us, this doctor was not only the best dressed but he also appeared immaculate. Having done some tailoring, I recognized high-quality, woolen herringbone tweed suits which looked like they had just left a tailor's pressing iron. Bright colors for menswear were not popular at the time. However, his clothing was colorful enough to be interesting but not drab enough to be dull. His outfits were coordinated, unwrinkled, and complete. Patients do notice missing buttons, mismatched clothing, spotted or wrinkled ties, and the like. Even if Dr. Meads had been up all night delivering babies or performing surgical duties, he had that "put-together look."

After the galloping dandruff episode, I was relieved that Dr. Stolberg did not refer to it. When he visited me, he simply ignored the matter. For the doctor who was recommended by a peer for his communication skills, I found him to be rather terse, stiff, and straight. During visitors' hours one evening, I was watching people making their way down the corridor from my wheelchair in the hall. Dr. Stolberg, still in his heavy winter coat, stopped to greet me as he went by. He asked how I was feeling. I replied, "I'm doing just fine, but you don't have all your buttons." His face had a quizzical look as he shoved his hand into his coat pocket, pulled out the missing coat button, and showed the button in his extended palm. Apparently, he discussed neurological and muscular functions with patients at length, but I don't recall hearing any other subjects or any humor. Granted, humor is not essential, but it certainly equals, "A little bit of sugar makes the medicine go down." On the professional level, without reservation I rank him and his associate, Dr. Deming, among the highest. Many thousands of times in the forty-some years since, I thank the powers that be for placing me in the Jackson County polio center. That rehabilitation team did everything possible to facilitate my recovery.

Now that I was more mobile, I visited some of the other patients. Among them, I met a former school mate who was recovering from back surgery. Over six feet in height, he had been the basketball team's star player. Because he was an upperclassman, I had known him only by watching basketball games. Now he was a man of the cloth, a minister with a fine sense of humor. Evidently his profession did not rule against card-playing because we played Canasta every spare hour afternoons and evenings until he was discharged. In fact, I played cards so much during that hospital stay that I haven't had the urge to play since. Anytime there were no prescribed routines and no visitors, each contacted the other one for a game. The Reverend was also permitted wheelchair privileges, so sometimes we gathered at the chart room for ice or conversation with the nurses when they weren't busy.

After visiting hours one evening, the Reverend and I were chatting by the chart room when a man ran into the room. He gasped at the nurse, "My wife is in a pickup truck in the parking lot just outside (the entrance to the stairs leading to the chart room.) She's in the front seat delivering a baby." The nurse took a quick look out the window and said, "Oh my God!" A doctor in street clothes walked past the chart room. The nurse grabbed him by the coattail and told him, "Come on!" On her way out of the room, she told the Reverend to phone someone for a gurney, a wheelchair, and help. The Reverend wheeled himself to the chart room phone and conveyed her messages.

Evidently word got through because almost before he replaced the phone, we saw a green-covered gurney being wheeled out by two, green-gowned-and-masked women. The doctor's back was toward us. When he turned sideways, he held an upended baby by the feet before he handed it off to the green-garbed assistants. They wrapped the baby, placed it on the gurney, and rushed it through the freezing rain into the hospital. When next seen, the doctor was helping the woman out of the truck's front seat into a wheelchair. Later, the nurse told us that the baby was fine, but it had to be placed in pediatrics because it had not been born in the hospital environment. For that reason, it could not be placed with the other babies in the nursery. For the same reason, the mother went into the women's section, not with the other nursing mothers. My only contribution to this momentous event was to stand by and answer aides when they asked where the charge nurse was and, "What was she doing out there?" in the snow and ice of the parking lot.

Most patients on our wing were considered serious, some improved so they could leave, a few died; but a few of us lingered longer than the others. A married couple in their fifties checked in about the same date as I. Both of them were seriously injured in an automobile accident on Christmas Eve.

Their arrival at the hospital was just a day before mine, but they remained on the critical list for a month or six weeks. Mrs. MacArthur, an energetic widow in her mid-fifties, also joined us on the wing late in December. I can't remember the nature of her injury, but she had a wonderful sense of humor. She was bedridden most of her stay, but since I had wheels, we had many fine visits. Eleanor followed me by a couple of days and she left about the same time as I did. But those of us who were mobile got to know others who visited or left before us. We became rather clannish and called ourselves "Members of Foote Hospital Spa."

Now I realize that after getting used to institutional food, it seems tasteless and monotonous. Someone in food service told me that most institutions rotate menus on a two-week basis. I began to long for variety. Probably more often than I realized, I voiced my longing for a hamburger smothered in onions and a chocolate milkshake. One Saturday, two separate couples brought me a hamburger with onions and a chocolate malted. Luckily, those thoughtful gifts were separated by a couple of hours, so I ate every gift with gusto. Never have I tasted better burgers and malts.

The aides, mostly young people in their late teens or early twenties, were especially helpful. Depending on the patient load, there were sometimes half a dozen on the day shift. These young people made life much pleasanter for those of us who had special needs. They greased the wheels so service was quick, pleasant, and seamless. In addition to making beds, helping us dress, and emptying bedpans; they adjusted beds, brought us objects we couldn't reach (like books, stationery or candy), covered us when we couldn't manage covers ourselves, and helped us navigate our wheelchairs. Just when it became apparent that most of them had significant others of the same sex eludes me. Neither Eleanor nor I were we surprised. It just seemed like a fact of life which didn't affect us one way or another.

These were some of the most caring people: they wanted to be needed; to serve them gave satisfaction. After they had completed their assignments, they often congregated in our room. This we encouraged by offerings of candy and other edibles. (One of the reasons the charge nurse listened on the intercom was to locate the aides when she needed them. Our room often held the answer.) We welcomed their visit because so often our own family was unable to visit. The aides brought us the news of the hospital as well as the news of the day. Most of them, when they had a day off, asked if we wanted them to do any shopping for us; was there anything we needed? This was a very special offer, indeed.

Another special memory is a regular evening aide who brought a trolley full of cold, fruit drinks after visiting hours were ended just before lights out. She was a short, heavyset, colored woman named Eleanor who always had a kind smile on her face. What I felt from her was like a mother's love when she came to my bed and asked, "What do you want, little one?" My request was always for apricot nectar, but she asked just in case I opted for another flavor. My choice was triggered by the memory of when I first had the tracheotomy, the first days I could swallow. During those days when I thirsted, I dreamed of mountains of icy apricot nectar, orange sherbet, and frozen orange juice.

A bedtime ritual then, which I doubt is performed now, occurred when it was time to make patients ready for bed and just before lights out. First, the nurse or aide straightened the patient's bed covers. Next, she stored wheelchairs in the hall so they wouldn't be stumbled over on the way to the bath. Then she stored books, gifts, etc. on the window sill. And the most pleasurable came last: the back rub. This was no slap-dash effort. Five minutes of relaxing massage and pleasant conversation made the prospect of long, dark hours more tolerable.

My roommate, Eleanor, and I had few evening visitors. Eleanor's home was in Cassopolis, a hundred miles from the hospital. Her husband was an active partner in a well-drilling business, a heavy labor-and-time-consuming business. Drilling a well in Michigan's winter weather meant long hours in the bitter cold. Wilbur did well if he could visit once during the week and once or twice on weekends. Making the trip after work and in unpredictable weather conditions worried everyone. When he was able to make the trip, he arrived long after visiting hours; often after midnight. The nurses understood this and made no objections.

My husband, Bill, had again taken on an evening job in addition to his daytime meatcutter's work, this time as bartender. The stated reason for the extra job was to save a down payment on a house. Thank goodness the March of Dimes Foundation underwrote all my medical and hospital expenses. Adding a housekeeper to our household expenses was not as great an expenditure as it might be today. Catherine received her room and board plus $15 a week, as I remember. We weren't aware that the Foundation might also have helped with the full-time housekeeper which would have made life much easier. Had I been able to continue my typing-at-home job, which ceased when I came down with polio, we could have managed on Bill's daytime job alone.

But the bartending job was in a tavern where he habitually spent the greater part of his off-the-job time. Working there permitted him to continue the social association and, at the same time, be paid. At least, I think he was paid. As long as he worked there (over a period of several years), no evidence of additional income surfaced until I figured our income tax. But I was in no position to confront.

One of my faculties which had been left intact was the libido. I longed for my husband's warm embraces and the release that intimacy would bring. Being viewed as an attractive person, one worthy of and attractive enough to love, was of deep concern. With my new mobility and the nurse's permission to go where there were no RIs, Bill and I wandered to the opposite end of the hall where there was a round, solarium-type room with padded benches. When Bill did arrive, it was late, after he had closed the bar (closing time was 2 a.m.). We went down to the solarium. There were no visitors at this late hour. One inhabitant, a male aide, slept on the padded surface until the nurse needed him. He was the one with the strong back; available when patients needed to be lifted. Nurse knew where he was. He must have been playing possum because, by the time we had selected the most isolated place, he had quietly left the area. The loving was very special, very tender. It left me stronger to meet whatever challenge the next day offered.

We had a new evening charge nurse, Miss Shirl Lautenbach, fresh from the Army. She wore an unusual nursing cap, unique in that it laced up the back. Miss Lautenbach was pretty, petite, and forceful. When visitors lingered more than ten minutes past evening visiting hours, she stood at the end of the hall, left hand on her hip, right hand and index finger pointed at the door as she commanded, "Visitors OUT!" And out they went! That gruff exterior shielded a warm and sympathetic individual. The day I was discharged, Shirl said to me, "If you ever need help, just call me." Her words echoed in my ears later when, in desperation, I called her.

At first, Catherine our housekeeper, had matters well in hand. From Bill and my mother, I heard nothing but good reports. Naturally I thought often about home. But thinking of home and children sharpened the already keen edge of my longing to hold my children, smell their child-baby smell, exchange wet kisses, and feel their warmth. While I was in the hospital they didn't come to visit. At Christmas time, the armslings frightened them. I was still wearing the same armsling arrangement when I stood up. The marvelous wheelchair with its overhead armslings was truly convenient, but it might also frighten them even more.

Part of the dilemma was solved by hospital policy: young children were not permitted to visit anyhow. Besides, I was at high risk for respiratory infections which they might inadvertently bring. Bill could have brought the girls to the hospital parking lot in the car and lingered by our first-floor window long enough for me to glimpse them. He didn't offer and I didn't ask. Nor did I talk with them on the phone because it would only have increased my restlessness. Had I not been kept busy with daily routines and buried myself in reading, playing canasta, and visiting other lonely patients, the waiting would have been even less bearable.

Almost as soon as we became roommates, Eleanor and I had discovered we both enjoyed reading. On one of his visits, "Doc" Lewis brought us a book describing recent research about a silver cup purportedly used by the disciples at the Last Supper. Photographs of the cup showed the bas-relief image of a clean-shaven, short-haired Jesus whose hair was cut straight across the forehead, like "bangs." The unfamiliar representation of such a prominent figure triggered our interest. Eleanor was an excellent reader who could hold a heavy book, such as this one (and other "proper" or hardbound books as well). Now that I had the wheelchair with the lap board, I might have handled the heavier books. But paperbacks were far easier to manage. By myself, I read paperbacks. When Eleanor and I were whiling away the long evenings, she read from the larger tomes. And many are the evenings we "whiled."

Almost always, after scheduled lights out, Eleanor read to us an hour or two past midnight. By that time we knew whether our husbands would visit. After that question was answered, we could settle ourselves to sleep. For the first time we appreciated the advantage of being housed at the end of the hall. Our reading and talking after visiting hours in this location was less apt to disturb other patients. After the rest of the patients had been tucked in for the night, the nurse pushed our door almost shut so we could amuse ourselves as late was we wished.

Sometimes she read, sometimes we just talked. We talked of families, husbands, hobbies, dreams of the future. We became very close friends. We also kept a bottle of wine in our "stash" (with the doctors' and nurses' knowledge). Every time I made a milestone or achieved a goal in physical therapy, we had a small "toddy" in celebration. We also paid the price of those who burn the midnight hours.

The price was collected early the following morning. Jimella, the maid, arrived before daylight to dry mop and then wet mop the floor. She was a wonderful tease. Right away she recognized that Eleanor was not a morning person. Eleanor wanted neither noise nor conversation until she had had her first cup of coffee. However, our room was first on Jimella's assignment because we were at the end of the hall. And Jimella's job started before breakfast or coffee was delivered. When that lady started with the dry mop, she made only swishing sounds. Once she started with the wet mop and pail, it was bang, bang, bang on Eleanor's metal bed frame until Eleanor shouted herself awake. At Eleanor's indignant reaction, Jimella bent over her mop pail panting with laughter. Then we all had a good laugh. Eleanor would admit that she "had been had" and proceed more graciously into the day.

On the last day of Jimella's work week, we asked her what she was going to fix for Sunday dinner. She always answered, "chicken." Soon we teased her about liking nothing but chicken. Not a year afterward, I found out that Jimella died of cancer of the stomach.

Eleanor, the evening aide who distributed liquid refreshments, also had her problems which she never permitted to surface on the job. This lady worked the evening shift so she could take care of her 300-pound, paralyzed mother during the day. What big hearts and shared humor covered these women's heavy burdens.

Student nurses and nurses' aides rotated through our area carrying out their respective duties. Soon their faces, names, and voices became familiar. They knew that we enjoyed their company. They also knew we had a cache of tasty edibles to which they were welcome. Sometimes their visits were professional, carrying out the charge nurse's directives. Other times they just dropped in when they had a moment to spare. After sharing classes and work assignments, these people had formed a rather cohesive group. They had developed a camaraderie that extended beyond working hours into recreational activities as well.

I did a double-take one evening during visiting hours. While I was sitting in my wheelchair watching other people's visitors pass down the hall, I was surprised to see a familiar face. But the person was not dressed as an aide. Instead of the tailored uniform, my impression remains one of many white ruffles. She was about my height, rather stockily built, and moved with ease and quickness. She said, "I'm Liz. I came to visit you." This astounded me because she had been in and out of our room several times during the day shift. Now she was back to visit at seven in the evening! Also, it was evident that she had made a special effort to dress up. For me! I hadn't known her name before, but she gave me the full moniker and said she had been in my high school class twelve years ago. In school, we were sorted into session rooms and seated alphabetically. With over 350 in the class and her surname nowhere near mine, I wasn't too embarrassed that I didn't remember her. We didn't have a lot to talk about after those few words. But I remembered to thank her for coming to visit. I didn't know that after I had left the hospital, we would meet again under dramatically different conditions.

After Bill and I had met a few times in the solarium, Dr. Meads suggested maybe it was time I had a "pass." Anything that goes on in their area of the hospital nurses know about. And what the nurse knows, she tells the doctor. So I am sure Dr. Meads knew Bill and I had rendezvoused. "Just what is a pass?" I asked. "Oh, you can go out a couple of hours in the evening about visitors' time. Get you used to being outside the hospital. But dress warmly," was his explanation.

I called Bill to tell him. He was able to take off from his evening shift at the tavern that night so we could use the pass. When he arrived, I was completely dressed. I even wore shoes! My winter coat and a kerchief for my head were handy. He helped me down the stairs to the car. Luckily he had found a parking spot near the door. He headed the car toward the tavern where he worked. It was located near the beginning of Skid Row. Around the corner from the tavern was the entrance to an upstairs hotel. This was no residential hotel. It was a location where people "turned tricks." Married women are not supposed to know these things, but because of Bill's employment in the area, I did. However, the hotel was located close to the hospital and it afforded the privacy we wanted and needed.

The desk clerk must have been confused when we signed in. I could picture him wondering, "How was the feeble-looking, shuffling, hooker with the broken arms able to attract a John?" But I was more interested in being alone with my husband than I was concerned about a desk clerk's opinion. Two or three hours later we returned to the hospital, quiet but comfortable with ourselves and one another.

During the next month, Dr. Meads let me have one or two more evening passes. Then he suggested I try going out for an entire day during a weekend, so I could go home and see what it looked like. Late in April I survived the one-day-home visit. Moderate weather had announced the arrival of spring. Believing that the worst of the winter was over, both doctors and Miss Holton agreed that I could plan to go home early in May provided I had a housekeeper. Eleanor, my roommate, had already left as had the other three long-term residents of "Foote Hospital Spa." So for a second time, my discharge from hospital was arranged.

The wonderful wheelchair with overhead armslings and lap board went home with me. Miss Holton said she and the doctors wanted me to have it as long as I needed to use it. Probably they imagined the same kind of scene I did: home life as a continuation of hospital routine. The surroundings would be different, my activities would remain much the same, but Catherine would be in charge. However, instead of the assistance I had received from hospital staff, Catherine would help me. As in the hospital, I would spend the greater part of the day in the wheelchair with daily visits to Physical Therapy, but I would not yet shoulder the responsibilities of child-rearing and homemaking.

On a glorious Sunday morning in May, Bill brought me home. I could smell the grass, iris were ready to bloom, trees showed big buds, and the air smelled of growing things. He brought me, my suitcase, and the wheelchair into the house. While Catherine had her usual day off, Bill's sister, Frances, had taken over. But Frances had to leave as soon as Bill and I arrived from the hospital. That left just the four of us: Bill, me, and the two girls. Together we ate the lunch Catherine had prepared the day before. Eating a meal with Bill and the children for the first time since Christmas was a joy. As soon as he finished eating, Bill left to go to his Sunday afternoon shift at the tavern. I was alone with the girls from early afternoon until the bar closed after midnight. That's when reality set in.

However, this was the weekend. Catherine had earned her agreed-upon time off. In her absence, Frances, my sister-in-law had stayed until I appeared. Like other members of my husband's family, she was a workaholic. During the week she worked a high-stress job in a factory; on weekends she went home to work on the farm. Only lately I found that the children pulled every stunt they could on Frances while she stayed with them. Although they were only two and five years old, when they made up their minds, they could be hellions. I can understand their thinking. Their mother had gone who knew where, they had had a succession of baby-sitters and housekeepers—some familiar, but most of them odd. Now the family had moved into an unfamiliar town with yet another housekeeper. One child had changed schools and both had to make all new friends. Life must have seemed very precarious to them. They probably figured, when in doubt, stir up a disturbance.

Apparently, at the time, everyone thought that once I was out of the hospital, I was cured. Everything would return to normal or to the way it had been. I hadn't given it much thought. Like the ostrich, I had buried myself trying to get well enough to return home while ignoring the reality of home. If I thought about it at all, I assumed that getting over polio would be like getting over a cold or the flu. In a few days—at most a couple of weeks—I would be as good as new. The doctors had warned me that it might take a matter of years, but I had dismissed it from my mind.

However, in the meantime, I had two very active youngsters and a housekeeper who did not return early evening as expected. In fact, she didn't return that night. Bill would not be home until after midnight. I can't remember what we ate for supper, only that we ate. If there was something already fixed in the refrigerator, that could have been it. If not, we ate "bread-and-with-it." I was unable to cut, slice, or butter bread, but Cynthia could spread peanut butter and jam which was always acceptable. Fortunately, she could also handle a milk bottle. Glass or cardboard, I had not the strength to grasp it. Somehow we got through the evening and I put the girls to bed. I couldn't lift Linda into her child's bed, so I told her to hang on around my neck and I lifted her that way. Because I couldn't push a safety pin through her diapers either, I tied them where the pins should have been. Between us, we got the job done.

Knowing that the next day, Monday, Bill would work his 8-5 job (where store policy required a clean, white shirt), I checked the closet. No clean, white, ironed shirts. The basket offered clean laundry, but no ironed shirts. Assembling the ironing board and iron required many pauses for rest. Lifting the iron brought searing pain, but I managed to smooth out the collar, fronts, and cuffs—the parts of a shirt that would show around his store apron. Then I collapsed in bed.

Allowing myself to go to sleep was still an act of faith. When I permitted myself to think about it, I wondered if I would remember to breathe once I fell asleep. But, this time I was so worn out I slept almost instantly. In fact, I slept so well, I didn't even awaken when Bill came to bed after closing the tavern.

Fortunately, Catherine returned the next day, hangover and all. She recited some unbelievable story about her boyfriend, Hermie, leaving her where she couldn't find a phone. Too desperate and dependent upon her, I didn't press the issue. From then on, whenever she left for her weekend sallies, I never felt sure of her return. This happened enough times that we finally had to dispense with her services. But for the time being, she stayed with us and very good help she was while she remained sober.

In her defense, Catherine was a practical, frugal, and wonderful cook. She made biscuits that would float in the sky. Her baked beans were one of Linda's favorites. Linda would beg Catherine to make "Beanos." And Catherine made them every week or so. Catherine joined the ranks of those openly viewing me with suspicion because I either could not or would not pitch in and work. She assisted me when need forced me to ask, but she made it clear that technically this was not part of her job description.

Everyone seemed to think I was goofing off. God knows, had I been able to do more or love more, I would have done so without hesitation. I longed to hold and roughhouse with my children as I used to do. As it was, I couldn't comb or wash their hair, fix much food, clean house, or do laundry. In fact, for some time, I often didn't have enough strength left to raise either arm to wash my own face, comb my hair or brush my teeth. In between housekeepers, there were days when I didn't get washed, brushed, or cleaned. When Catherine was gone, the girls and I ate much of our food with our hands because I couldn't butter bread or cut food.

The living quarters we rented just before Christmas were part of a two-bedroom bungalow we shared with the owner, Mr. Phil. We were fortunate to find a rental within our means because reasonably priced rentals were very scarce then, as they are now. The division of the available room contributed to an interesting situation. Mr. Phil, a widower of Catherine's age or older, retained one bedroom for himself. We shared the bath, the kitchen facilities, and the use of the basement where our laundry equipment was located. He spent most of his waking hours either in the full basement or, in pleasant weather, on the back porch or in the backyard. This arrangement lasted for the better part of nine months.

To get from his bedroom to the back porch or to the bath, Mr. Phil had to pass through the kitchen. At first Catherine declared (more than once and with great fervor) that Mr. Phil had pinched her behind when she was cooking at the stove. Mr. Phil denied this vehemently. In his own defense, he maintained that she had been trying to flirt with him to get his attention. She, of course, denied his accusation. Next, Mr. Phil accused Catherine of stealing one of his saucepans. She adamantly denied the theft while pointing out that she had no need to steal saucepans because we had several. When the weather was warm enough for Mr. Phil and me to sit on the back porch while the children were sleeping and Catherine had been gone several weeks, he admitted he had found the missing pan. It was in the backyard where he had left it with scraps for the dog he often fed.

While Catherine was still with us, I managed to keep the car. This took some courage because I wasn't sure I could drive a standard shift with my left hand. The right hand still hung in a sling and, to this day, there is no extension forward. In the Navy we indicated our termination with the phrase, "Rain, snow, s—t, hail or shine!" Not only was I insistent that I wanted the use of the car, but I was equally certain that I could drive it. Once I reached through the D-ring of the steering wheel with my left hand to shift, it was fairly simple. That meant that when I had use of the car, I could drive myself to physical therapy. I didn't have to take the bus.

After being home a few weeks, cabin fever set in. I felt as though I would explode if I didn't get out of the house for something other than therapy. It was not yet the sticky, humid, hot Michigan summer and the weather was pleasant and inviting. The idea of a picnic kept running through my mind. How much fun for the girls and me to have an afternoon picnic in the park. Although Bill never let us go hungry, nether did we have ready-made picnic fare. Besides, preparing such food would have dissipated whatever energy I had. Peanut-butter sandwiches and one bottle of pop would have to do. Cynthia was able to make and cut two sandwiches that we put in a bag. I found a bottle opener and we climbed into the car. One of the city's most beautiful parks was only a mile distant. Too early for picnic tables, so we sat on the grass with our backs against a tree to eat our peanut butter sandwiches and share a bottle of warm pop. A humble picnic it was, but satisfying. It fulfilled my need to get out of the house, to do something different and memorable with the children.

One of my worst fears (something would happen to the girls that I would be unable to cope with) coincided with the date Cynthia's school let out. The youngster started showing signs of fever and weakness. Very soon, she was flushed, burning with fever, and almost comatose. She neither moved nor talked. All I could do was sponge her with cool water to try to bring her fever down. Although her symptoms didn't seem to resemble the onset of polio, it was still a possibility. In desperation I called Dr. Meads to report the symptoms. He stopped by to look at her an hour later after office hours. He couldn't make a diagnosis because she wasn't coughing, vomiting, or showing signs of skin eruptions. When he left he said, "Call me when anything else happens."

An hour or so later, Cynthia had a heavy nosebleed. Fortunately, I was able to stop it. Deeply worried, I reported the latest event to the doctor. He laughed and said, "Don't worry. It's only measles. Keep her quiet and in the dark as much as you can. I'll stop by tomorrow and give Linda shot which may prevent her from getting them." As good as his word, the next day he gave Linda a shot. Although she did catch the measles, it was a light case of the three-day variety. However, when Dr. Meads saw Cynthia again, he said she had the worst case of German measles he had seen in thirty years. Thanks to my good friend, the children were safe.

After Cynthia and Linda had recovered from their respective maladies, I needed to take them downtown for something. I don't remember why, but I do know that the car was not available. What is significant is that although I had been taking the bus regularly to physical therapy, this was the first time we three had ever taken public transportation. The bus stopped only half a block from our house. Three of us and another couple waited there for it.

The bus, when it came, was old, hot, noisy, and belched lots of black exhaust. Cynthia climbed up the steps without hesitation. However, my 2-1/2 year old was terrified. I still carried both arms in slings, so I could do little except nudge her forward and encourage her with words. When I pushed, she spread-eagled her arms and legs against the door and screamed at the top of her voice. The driver looked at me in amazement. Sizing up the situation, the man behind me asked, "Lady, do you want this child on the bus?" When I nodded, he picked up the screaming, kicking child and set her firmly on the floor of the bus. When she realized she was going to have to ride regardless of the noise and fumes, she sat down with a scowl. All during the fifteen-minute ride she sat sulking, arms folded, looking like an angry pigeon with ruffled feathers who is about ready to pounce.

After word got round that I was home from the hospital, we were invited out by Bill's co-workers. Because after a while sitting up was uncomfortable, I asked if anyone minded if I laid down on the floor. No one objected. However, either they thought it odd or else Bill was embarrassed by his wife's behavior because we were seldom invited back.

Dad visited us at Mr. Phil's house several times. Toward the end of summer, he loaned us a thousand dollars to make a down payment on a place of our own. Considering all the medical expenses he had with my stepmother's advanced cancer, he must have mortgaged both body and soul to give us the money. In spite of Bill's second job at the tavern, the additional expense of a housekeeper made it impossible to accumulate money for a down payment. It is possible that the March of Dimes might have helped us with the expense of a home-care person, but we didn't know, and we were too grateful for the immense expense already underwritten by them to ask. Bill's second job, taken for the expressed purpose of saving for a house payment, seemed to be on a par with chicken soup: it might have helped, but in reality, we seemed no further ahead. On the other hand, his long hours away from home made for a very lonely life, one in which neither I nor the children saw very much of him awake.

Just how my dad was able to make the loan remains a mystery. My best guess is that somehow he borrowed it in the hope that having our own living quarters would make our lives pleasanter. We wouldn't have to share rather limited space with the owner—a someone else who always seemed to clash head-on with any housekeeping person we were able to hire. Being a homebody himself, possibly dad thought

Bill would concentrate on working one job and put leftover energy into fixing up a home of his own.

Even with the down payment, a first home in our financial situation would necessarily be a fixer-upper. Although World War II had ended seven years before, housing had been scarce even before the war. The building industry was booming, but it hadn't caught up with the demand created by veterans and their families. What we selected within our price range that fall was a two-story, older, frame house with two big bedrooms upstairs. Downstairs included living room, dining room, a small den or bedroom with access to the basement, and a bath off the kitchen. Houses in this part of town were built mostly in the late 1890s or early 1900s, so a good guess would be that the bath off the kitchen was accomplished by turning what once was a pantry into the bath. The coal furnace in the old dirt basement was usable, the plumbing and electric were passable. The whole house needed a lot of cleaning and TLC (tender loving care). Although there was no garage, the deep lot gave us a good-sized back yard. On the plus side were wonderful neighbors, reasonable access to an elementary school, and mass transit only half a block away.

Another advantage was that Catherine had returned (for the third or fourth time) in time to help us move. Bill took his vacation to improve the kitchen. I doubt that he washed the walls before he painted. With his background as an experienced spray painter (of enamel), he decided to spray the kitchen ceiling and walls with high-gloss enamel. The color he chose was red — checkerboard red. It was my job to mask cupboards and windows with paper so he could spray around them. He had brought a huge roll of butcher paper for the masking process. When he finished an area, I was to clean up the spills.

After trying for an hour to be helpful, I was in misery from the pain in my back, arms, and shoulders. I sat on top of the two-foot-high wooden-centered roll of paper and cried. That roll of paper and the floor were the only places to sit. I cried from pain and frustration. From Bill's standpoint, he thought that if he could take his vacation to prepare the house for occupancy, the least I could do was help with the painting. Finally, in misery and anger, I shouted, "I'll bet you wish the old bitch had died."

Next on the fix-up agenda was the kitchen floor. Bill decided to use 9-inch squares of linoleum, alternating in red and black. The floor looked like a checkerboard. Fortunately, the white-enameled, metal cupboards were in good condition. Had it not been for the white sink and cupboards, the kitchen would have been darker and weirder than it already was. Luckily, Catherine stayed a few weeks after we moved so we were fairly well settled before she left permanently. Then I was totally on my own.

Several items were missing that would have made life on my own a whole lot easier. The wonderful wheelchair had been returned almost immediately because Mr. Phil's house was not "accessible." That is, the doorways were not wide enough and it wasn't possible for me to get in and out of it on my own. Neither Mr. Phil's house nor this one had 220-volt service, so the electric stove and dryer had to be disposed of. In between the move from Mr. Phil's house and our new home, the mangle or ironer had disappeared also. It had been a godsend at Mr. Phil's . Many times, when the housekeeper was absent, I spent evenings after the children were asleep in the basement with Mr. Phil. We had an arrangement whereby I washed the clothes, he hung them up and took them down. In return, I did his ironing on the mangle. Ironing by hand was still such torture. For a wife whose husband wore six or seven starched white shirts and four or five wash uniform pants a week, ironing was a project where a mangle was magic. This was only one of many reasons a dependable housekeeper would have been so appreciated.

Now that we were moved in, Bill went back to working his second job. We saw him briefly at breakfast (he was definitely not a morning person). If we saw him for supper, it was briefly in passing on his way to the tavern job. He came home after closing, long after we were in bed. Sometimes he spent his day or half day off around the house. More often he went to the farm to check on his folks. One of his half days off, he got in the car to run an errand. I asked if we could ride along. When asked why he always had to leave on his day off, he replied, "The children make me nervous." Years later Cynthia offered me insight into the situation. She recalled that there was a wooded area nearby where she and other youngsters used to catch small grass snakes. She kept her snakes in glass jars. She also knew that snakes (living or dead, dangerous or otherwise) frightened her father. Every once in a while she put a jar with a live snake in his car. Forty-odd years later she admitted, "I used to put the grass snakes in his car. Sure I made him nervous." The Curey humor could be a bit odd at times.

Our first winter in the new-old house turned bitter cold. Bill loaded the furnace and banked the fire in the morning. By afternoon, the house was chilly. By evening I was in the basement throwing coal into the furnace piece-by-piece trying to keep the place warm. I couldn't hold a shovel and there was no way I could heave a shovelful of coal. But somehow we managed.

My neighbors were concerned and helpful. When Catherine left, one of them offered to watch Linda for the two hours it took to go to physical therapy three times a week.

This Christmas I was better prepared for the holidays. Knowing that shopping in the crowded stores and carrying bundles was not for me, I relied on my handy, free, Sears catalog. I could read product descriptions and compare them as much as I pleased. All I had to do after I placed the order was make one trip to the store to pay for it. Then I could use the car to pick up the entire order from the loading dock. I've relied on this system frequently ever since.

After we had lived in the house about a year, the neighbor who had offered to watch Linda came for a visit one afternoon. Finally she came to the point of the visit. She and the neighbors would like to buy me a dress. They assumed we were too poor to afford a dress because they had seen me only in slacks and long-sleeved blouses. Then I explained to her that Miss Holton had advised that for a year or two, I should keep arms and legs covered to protect myself from the sun. It was not to protect from skin cancer, it was to avoid kidney problems. The therapist's explanation was that the pigmentation of the skin had been affected by polio so the skin did not protect me. The sun's rays could affect the kidneys. We both laughed over the misunderstanding. What kindness the neighbors showed.

Another neighbor, "Piney," lived down the block at the edge of a very busy intersection. I never knew whether it was a nickname because she grew dozens of peony bushes or because the pronunciation of her Russian name sounded like that. Anyway, old Piney was described as one who hated children; she didn't want to be bothered by them. But every time I turned my back in good weather, Linda ran away from the perimeter of our lot. One busy noontime Piney came puffing up to my door to tell me in broken English that Linda was trying to cross the busy intersection in front of Piney's house. Linda may owe her undamaged body to that kind woman.

Part Two

Change for the better often comes from unexpected directions. For instance, never did it occur to me the IRS would insist that we arrange to pay back taxes immediately. But this demand is the firecracker which changed my outlook and lifestyle. When the previous year's tax was due, I was in the middle of my hospital stay—not at home to figure our tax as I usually did. Keeping focused on the daily hospital routine had helped me remain reasonably calm. Income tax hadn't yet registered on my radar screen. I was just trying to settle into the routine of being home. The fact that two years' taxes were overdue shocked me. But the IRS man truly startled me with the blunt statement, "Either pay up or we'll take your home."

"Either" meant we must begin making substantial and regular payments on the debt. "Or" promised that if the debt were not attended to, we would lose our home.

Housing had been appallingly scarce for several years. Now, cold fear of losing our home forced me to face alternatives—most of them not pleasant. To ignore the IRS position meant more than the loss of the house. It also meant losing what we had paid on the mortgage and ruining our credit rating. Available housing had not caught up with demand since before World War II. Returning veterans like us in 1954, who were starting families of their own, were vying for their own premises. Although Bill paid the necessities, he refused to increase withholding or make IRS payments. We never even considered asking our families for assistance. So, that left the option of finding additional income to satisfy the IRS.

Marketable skills I knew I had, but just living day-to-day, minding the house and children and fighting 'cabin fever' sapped my available energy. The only person I consulted about returning to work was my physical therapist whom I still saw three times a week. She didn't tell me, "No." But she did say, "If you will rest at least twenty minutes before you get too tired, you can possibly extend your day up to two hours."

Surprise! My first application proved successful! The local telephone company hired me for a top clerical position. Fortunately, the company knew my work history because I had worked there before I enlisted in the Navy (WAVES) in 1944. And being a veteran gave an applicant extra points.

When I didn't have to use the right hand to write, I still carried the arm in a sling to keep the weight (and pain) off the right shoulder. But that didn't seem to faze my employer.

Bill found a baby sitter, a mature woman he knew from the bar where he worked nights. She seemed pleasant, clean, and liked children. Cynthia now seven, was in first grade most of the day. But the younger, Linda, an active almost five-year-old, needed watching. For me, starting to work an 8-hour day (plus public transportation) was as difficult as weaning myself from the breathing machine. Had it not been for the fascination of the job and the assurance that the effort would help secure our home, working would have exceeded my endurance.

Dealing with tired children who must be fed, cuddled, bathed and read to before bedtime left me utterly exhausted. My prayer was for patience to see me through until their bedtime. After that, it was my time—time to fill the claw foot bathtub with warm water, grab a paper-back book, and soak away the pain and fatigue. Pain medication was not considered at the time—not even an aspirin.

Thursday was payday on the new job—the day when the eagle screamed. My first check made me exuberant. The second check made a payment to the baby sitter and the IRS. But the third was the last check. Not because I couldn't do the work. The real reason for quitting was because I learned the baby sitter took Linda to Skid Row bars where she sold her crocheting. That kind of baby sitting was not acceptable.

Leaving my new job, the friends I had known and the new ones I had made, was more hurtful than the loss of income. The flip side was new knowledge—the assurance that with dependable child care, working was possible.

In the aftermath of that fiasco, I became better acquainted with my neighbor, Leila Boyer, who lived just two houses away. She was a widow who did laundry to support herself and her two teenage children. She was also the kindly person who earlier, on behalf of the neighborhood, had offered to buy me a dress if I didn't have one. But it still came as a pleasant surprise that Leila was interested in looking after my two. She would take charge of Linda who was not yet in school, see Cynthia off to school in the morning when I caught the bus to work, and look after both girls in the after school time. We made a mutually acceptable agreement which lasted several months until I was more established.

Undaunted by my first failure, I applied to the gas-and-light utility. This time, a rigorous physical exam was required. My right arm still carried in a sling and the brighter scar at the base of my neck from the tracheotomy made it impossible to present myself as a normal, healthy applicant. The stiff-and-starch nurse readied me for the doctor. Laid out on the exam table, I wore nothing but a white sheet (not unusual under the circumstances). While we waited for the doctor, I said to her, "All I need is a white lily in my hand."

With her steely eyes fixed on me, she answered with her British accent, "That's not necessary." Her starched uniform rustled as she walked out of the room and the doctor entered. A pleasant, elderly man, he must have been generous in his report because I was hired.

Not only was I hired, but I was also assured that I would be assigned to "the school" training section for six months at the generous sum of $50 a week (this was an unheard-of starting wage in 1954). Unsaid was that six months was also the probation period. But the "perks" of the probation period truly surprised me: Blue Cross insurance for the family, paid holidays (plus days for sick leave) and the specific understanding that I would not be "docked" for the three times a week (about an hour each) it took for me to attend prescribed, ongoing, physical therapy.

In the school department, new hires were trained in the letter-and-form styles used by the various departments. This is where my marketable skills and past experience paid off. I drew on English, high school German and Latin classes for grammar and syntax; from previous employers I had experience in transcribing voice dictation, and the Navy had reinforced transcription of Morse code and drilled me on typing numbers accurately. With this background, I could be a copy typist, transcriptionist or a statistical typist. And I enjoyed these assignments. So maybe the previous job was not for me; perhaps it was just a warm-up for this wonderful opportunity.

Adapting to the new office routine was smoothed by the employer's understanding of a typist's equipment needs. I was encouraged to select a typing chair from the available styles. The chair was adjusted to fit me. It was raised until I sat high enough that my arms slanted down; I didn't have to hold them in a raised position and pound on the keys as required by manual machines. Stroking electric keys took less energy than punching the manual machine keys. (The typewriters were all IBM electric's—not terribly common at the time).

I worked my way through the school's sample book and soon was assigned some transcription. To be "usable," work had to conform to several rules:

1. No erasures permitted on letterhead.
2. No errors allowed in spelling or grammar.
3. No changes made in the dictator's dictation.

Halfway through the six months' school, I was assigned to a small transcription department comprised of six typists and a checker. The checker proofread our work for accuracy and correctness. If she found errors or omissions, the work was redone and evaluated again.

This was my graduation day! I had passed probation and was now a full-fledged, full-time employee with all the accompanying perks. Also, I was again able to make regular contributions to reduce the back income tax we owed. What a relief that was!

Sitting in one place to type took less energy than chasing a toddler, so I began to have more energy. The girls found our new routine pleasant. They enjoyed the new activities which came from my having more energy and a little more spending money.

After graduation with its welcome monetary increase, moving my typing equipment from the huge room, which housed nearly a hundred typists, proved to be an eye-opener. A fork-lift truck came up the elevator onto our floor, lumbered into the huge typing room, down the alley between the desks, and picked up my desk with my chair stacked on top. Once loaded, the truck backed out of the alley, out of the typing room, and deposited desk and chair in the smaller, 7-person department. No need to fit myself to another chair or learn where materials were located in this desk. The equipment, adjusted to my needs while in the school department, came with me to this new assignment.

I truly enjoyed the work. It lifted me out of my surroundings and away from my problems. True, it was a strict office. One was always early because the typewriters liked to be turned on and warmed up ten minutes before use. As soon as work began, time flew so fast that the next time I looked, the clock registered 10 o'clock when everyone on that floor took a 15 minute break. Noon was the next time I came up for air. Even if I ate lunch at my desk, I went out for a walk before resuming work at 1 o'clock. Soon I made friends to socialize with at lunch. This was a great step because, for quite some time, I had only my children to talk with at home. Talking with people my own age again was indeed a pleasant change.

In the mid-1950s, strict offices had dress-and-grooming requirements. Females wore dresses with skirts below the knee. Although short sleeves were tolerated, sleeveless dresses or spaghetti straps were not. Skin colored hose accompanied sensible walking shoes. One who appeared for work without hose or wearing spaghetti straps was directed to go home and return in proper attire—or not at all. Most employees walked or rode the bus to work. Few drove cars.

Bill still brought the groceries, stoked the furnace, ate an occasional meal long after the children's bedtime, slept and was gone before we were awake. Occasionally, he took us to his parents' farm on a Sunday afternoon. For the most part, we saw very little of him.

Months passed bringing relief from the IRS debt. This, in time, built up my self-assurance. Earlier in our marriage, requests to my husband for socializing or doing activities outside the home had created a tumultuous atmosphere. Now I started to feel the stirrings of self-reliance. In fact, I began to make demands.

We soon reached an impasse. I pleaded that we go to marriage counseling. At the first appointment, he backed out. I had thought continuing to go would demonstrate my intent to try to work things out. Evidently I was mistaken. Bill's reply was, "There's no reason for me to go. You've already told the counselor that it's all my fault and he wouldn't listen to me. So I'm not going." Not too long after that, the marriage ended in divorce because he continued to refuse to go to counseling or to modify his views on socializing.

Having been told before I left the hospital that anybody who had bulbar polio died soon after, I was eager to be close to a blood relative should I not be around to rear the children. When my mother and stepfather (the "the elders") learned of the impending divorce, they confided that they wanted to sell their home in a rather undesirable neighborhood. They suggested that, together, we buy a home and split expenses 50-50. I would use my GI loan application because my stepfather's health and age would probably be a deterrent to his getting a loan.

Although I wanted and needed a closer or blood relationship to help shelter the girls, this was not designed to be a full-time baby sitting job for mother. Cynthia was in school full-time and Linda was now in an all-day preschool where she learned to be more self-sufficient. The teacher picked her up in his small bus about 8 o'clock in the morning and delivered her home about 4:30. Mother would care for them a half hour in the morning and shortly longer in the afternoon. The arrangement seemed satisfactory to her. The plan sounded logical and reasonable. It also gave me reassurance about the girls' future should something happen to me.

So, I sold our first home and derived from the sale about the same amount as the down payment on our first home, the $1,000 my father had loaned us. But before my loan application for a larger house was even considered, the elders surprised me with the information that they had purchased a home that would fit us all. Maybe it wasn't according to the plan, but the neighborhood seemed pleasant, the school was excellent, and both school and my employment were within walking distance. Only that first change in plan should have been a red flag.

What again caught my undivided attention was that, so far as mother's judgment was concerned, Linda could do nothing right and Cynthia could do no wrong. Linda was born left-handed and no one, until now, had tried to make her switch. At mealtime, mother kept nagging at her, fussing, and threatening until Linda (as I remember doing in my highchair when under attack) spilled her food all over. And Linda, now fifty years later, remembers mother telling her, "If you're going to eat like a dog, eat with the dog!" Then, in despair, I watched mother put Linda's plate down by the dog's dish and Linda down beside it to eat.

These constant attacks destroyed my hard-won self-assurance and flung me back into the pattern of subordination. I felt like a vulnerable parasite who couldn't object for fear of losing the ground under me—more like a bug skewered on pin who could neither escape nor survive the environment. Why didn't I object to this? I was reduced to a quivering child again—unable to fight the greater power. It was not MY house, I was so painfully reminded. I was not strong enough or ready to confront these two powerful adults who, under the guise of concern and affection, had made a plan to get the three of us out of our own home into this hell we were living through.

Fortunately, June brought summer vacation with it. Other relatives came to the rescue. The girls were invited to visit their uncles in Michigan and Kentucky. Linda, who dearly loved the farm, went to be with her paternal grand-parents. Bill saw his daughters infrequently, whenever it was convenient for all concerned. Although I missed my children, I was grateful that they were freed from the atmosphere that prevailed at mother's. I tried to lose myself in work, get away on weekends if I could, and stay out of her way as much as possible thinking a vacation would bring back some semblance of peace.

With the end of summer vacation came new disruptions. There still was no way to please mother. Weekends were horrendous because we couldn't escape her tirades. We three outcasts visited the uncle in Grand Rapids one weekend, my father in Detroit the next. The third weekend, Bill called and asked if we could meet to talk.

The girls and I met him after church on Sunday in a soda bar. After some small talk, he told us that while he was at work my stepfather had come with an offer. According to Bill's version of the meeting, the elders had two doctors who would certify as to my fitness and sanity. Then, if Bill would also certify, the elders would take care of the children in return for the money their father, Bill, paid for the upkeep of his daughters, as set down by the Court.

After hearing this offer, Bill said he was so angry, it took two of his burly co-workers to hold him. That account was verified by the strong-arm workers who held him as well as other workers present all of whom I soon got to know. I was shocked by this news, but I was even more surprised that Bill was speaking like a husband and father who cared about his family.

For several days I felt as if I were being stalked. Then, as I was walking home after work I met Marthana, a friend from working together in PTA activities. Marthana was also mother's (our) neighbor in our new living arrangement. The short version of what the neighbor told me was she had seen mother earlier in the day. Mother had said they were going to do something drastic to me that night. My friend wanted me to be aware and on my guard. In passing she also mentioned that her upstairs apartment was available.

After dark, when the dishes were done, we three adults sought the coolness of the screened porch. It was dark and the girls were already in bed. With little discussion, my stepfather ordered me to get out of the house right then! Without warning, he snatched my purse out of my hand! Minus my pocketbook, I had no money or checkbook—no resources. Marthana's warning must have alerted me to try to prepare for the worst. He refused to give it back.

There was no alternative except to try to force him to return it. In desperation I began screaming at the top of my voice, "Give me back my purse! Give me back my money!" Realizing that neighbors were also enjoying the coolness of their porches as well as our discussion, he finally did surrender it.

Clutching the purse tightly, I hurried back into the house and dialed Marthana's number. I asked her if that apartment upstairs was available. When the answer was affirmative, I asked if we could come over. Again, I got an okay. So I woke the girls, packed some dry duds for each one, another outfit for myself and we three proceeded through the darkness to the waiting apartment. So much for the assistance and loyalty of blood relatives. I should remember this in the future.

Family disagreements are complicated affairs, but I'll try to analyze this one. Before jumping into this new, combined family arrangement, we had formalized a plan: the bookkeeper (mother) would total all the house and food expenses then divide them by five (the five members of the household). I was responsible for three-fifths of the total expense. This covered me and the girls. The other two-fifths was the responsibility of the elders (also the owners of the house). Responsibility for day school fees for Linda or any other personal expenses for the girls and me was mine alone. That's how it was supposed to work, at least the way I understood it would work. Obviously, it didn't work and we moved on to other arrangements.

While the girls and I lived in Marthana's apartment, I went to work and they to their schools as usual. We felt safe and protected. The neighbor also took me to look at a small, two -bedroom bungalow for sale nearby that she had considered purchasing for her mother. It had what we needed and was located even nearer to school and work. So I bought it even though my furniture was all in mother's house.

We couldn't live in the new house without furniture. Getting the furniture from the bastion of the elders seemed impossible. Again Marthana came to the rescue. She picked me up from work during my lunch hour, took me to the meat market where my stepfather worked and coached me to keep saying in a loud voice in front of his co-workers, "The children need their heavy clothes, the weather is getting cold, they need a bed to sleep in."

After a few minutes of this, he hissed, "OK. They'll be there in a couple of days." Further, Marthana arranged for her housekeeper to clean the house before our furniture and possessions were delivered. Although money was tight, I was more than glad to pay the housekeeper who made the house sparkle. I'll never be able to repay Marthana for all her kindnesses.

I've tried to leave the past in the past, but I couldn't help wondering why the elders wanted us in their house when it seemed they only wanted Cynthia, not her sister. They weren't prepared for me to disobey nor did they anticipate that the knowledge of their deed would be the key to catapulting me onto my own. Another nudge identified.

But, I wasn't exactly on my own. My ex-husband, Bill, had acted like a concerned and loving father—he had helped protect us. Always the optimist, I persuaded myself that he had changed into the loving, concerned father I had envisioned. He had changed jobs during the year we were separated. For a time, this was a good influence. The other employees' families were loyal and good friends. He seemed changed in this warm, supportive community.

We married again! We invited his friends and their families to our new home for a small celebration. Cynthia asked to take some of the party fare to her fourth grade teacher who asked, "What was the occasion."

"My mother got married," Cynthia answered.

"Whom did she marry?" inquired the teacher.

"My father," was the straight faced answer. When Cynthia came home to relate this event, she was mystified that the teacher laughed and pounded on the desk.

What changes had occurred since the divorce and remarriage? Bill made more money. He also spent more money and spent it away from home. On the other hand, I had established myself as a good employee, was getting regular raises, had insurance for me and the girls, was getting stronger, and no longer had the regular physical therapy sessions or wore the arm sling. In short, to most people, I was a "passer," an able-bodied person. That totaled a lot of psychological progress.

One exception, the scar from the tracheotomy at the base of my throat, made of deep red, keloid scar tissue, resembled a worm. Adults didn't comment, but little children asked, "Why is that worm on your neck?" The appearance I could accept, but the area became so deeply itchy that I felt I wanted to claw at it.

I remembered Dr. Wencke's, "You'll be back when you feel better." (After the tracheotomy tube was no longer considered necessary, the tube had been removed but the incision was allowed to heal—not sewn shut—in case the hole had to be used again.)

My appointment with the doctor was on a Saturday morning and I could see no other patients waiting. His greeting, "Who are you?" surprised me.

"You just don't know me with my clothes on," was my answer. The last time I had seen him, I was wearing only a towel under the chest respirator. He had never seen me dressed or upright.

"Oh, now I know who you are," he joked. He suggested that I have some deep x-ray done to prevent flesh from growing under the scar and to cease exerting pressure against scar tissue. The scar tissue was not elastic; it didn't grow or expand. The treatment provided relief from the itching and discomfort.

Sometime later, I followed up on his suggestion to have a revision of the scar which should have been a Z-plastic surgery. The Z shape would better distribute the weight over the torso. The surgeon elected to perform the straight up-and-down incision. This left a larger scar. But when healed, the scar was smaller and ultimately faded to match my skin color.

This is about four years after the onset of polio—the point where I had probably maximum return of muscle use. The left arm, although not at former strength, did provide full range of motion. The right hand I could raise to shoulder height. The legs seemed untouched. So to all appearances, I was "normal."

I can't say our home life was normal because Bill was seldom home during waking hours. He had formed a very strong bond with the men he worked with. They worked long hours and they played long hours. Their work was a combination of stevedore and over-the-road driver. Usually about 4 a.m. they unloaded refrigerated, railroad cars packed with Armour's meat products (unloading often meant picking up a 200 pound side of beef off the floor), loaded their trucks, and were on the road by 8 a.m. Anywhere from 3:30-5:30 p.m. they returned their trucks and regrouped at the local tavern where they hung out until about midnight. Although technically they were limited to a maximum of 8 hours of driving per day, they all kept two sets of logs. In case they were stopped, the logs showing appropriate work and rest periods would be produced.

Over a period of years, short-changing the body of necessary sleep had made changes in Bill's personality. His demeanor was gruff, almost angry at home. It concerned me to hear him speak of other drivers he worked with "getting in the back of the truck and letting Benny drive." This strongly suggested taking "uppers" or Benedryl to stay awake.

After a year or so, I began to have pain which increased with time. Concentrating on work didn't ease the pain. Still, no pain medication was offered or available. In early spring, I checked in with the rehabilitation doctors who asked what I was doing. When I described my schedule, their brusque reply was, "Quit your job. Now!" Even though I realized this made me dependent again, I quit my job and Bill was the sole provider.

During the summer I had a chance to recuperate. No more the long days at work and sewing late into the night. By fall, I was looking for a part-time job to get back into the swing of things. I missed financial independence and the social interaction.

Rehabilitation was suggested as a source of providing training for less strenuous work—hopefully the social work in which I was interested. Rehab agreed to underwrite the cost of books and tuition for a year at the local junior college. During an interview with a civil service supervisor, I was assured that there would be an opening for someone with my background and an associate degree—the degree I would complete in June.

In another sector during this period, successful oil wells were being drilled in the area adjoining the plot of land owned by Bill and his brother. One of my part-time jobs had been for the CPA firm headed by the husband of my good neighbor Marthana. When my CPA boss learned of the nearness of successful wells, he assembled buyers interested in purchasing oil rights from us. As the wife of one of the sellers, I sat in the meeting. As an employee of the CPA firm, I typed copies of the purchase deed.

From this transaction, the sellers received substantial, up-front money and an overriding interest—income from the well without responsibility for drilling costs. This 40 acre plot was eligible for two tries or holes—one try per 20 acres. The first hole, a year later, came in dry. The second hole, two years after the first, was successful. In another year, drillers "hit" oil in my former mother-in-law's home area, "Right where the chicken coop ought to be!"

All this excitement brought new stresses. Bill continued his schedule of extended wakefulness and too little sleep. He became more jealous and controlling. Even so, I was surprised when his friends called me for a date. When I recounted the telephone calls and named his friends, he doubled up with laughter. Then I realized that he had set this up; he found it very amusing.

Finally I admitted to myself that I couldn't change him. But I could change myself. I could remove myself from the situation and divorce was the logical exit. I had been so pig-headed, so determined to make this second marriage to Bill work. It would have been reasonable that with the same two personalities, one could predict the same outcome. If the first divorce was hurtful, this one was bitter. The first time we divorced, the girls were 5 and 8. This time, they were 11 and 13. And this time they remembered more and were hurt more deeply.

Probably the incredible stress of potential oil well production had broken already fragile bonds. As the divorce proceeded, the house had to be sold. Although the deed of ownership was in my name, the fallout of the divorce was that we split everything half-and-half. But some angel was looking over my shoulder when my lawyer got wind of the fact that Bill was not including his overriding oil rights in the division of property agreement. It still took three years before the well was producing oil or distributing money. In the meantime, I was dependent upon working for an irascible boss in a field I didn't care for. But we gals had a place to live and we ate well.

June came and with it the associate degree, honor status, but no civil service job was available. More importantly, the divorce was final which meant a full-time job was imperative. The civil service job description now called for a bachelor's but preferred a master's degree. Part-time employment had supplemented our diminished income this far. But other job prospects with civil service or elsewhere were dim at the present. Rehab had declined to underwrite any further education because to go forward with my program would have meant relocating to a college 45 miles away. What I needed now, right now, was a job which would feed us and ensure a place to live.

Although it was neither civil service nor social work, I settled for working in an insurance office where I took over most of the auto claims and became office manager. At home, I had a small transcription business. Through a friend I was introduced to a local millionaire who needed transcription and typing done. He delivered the dictation, I kept track of my time, and he paid me by the hour. Evidently he was satisfied with the work because he often gave me directions to, "Type it, sign it and send it." He also brought me four other manufacturers' representatives as clients who used this "drop off" transcription service. At one time, I had twenty letterheads showing the different companies these representatives worked for. Between these two pursuits, we weren't rich but we were secure.

One day I met my next-door neighbor, who kept close track of what went on in the neighborhood. I asked her what she thought of all the coming and going which accompanied the typing service. She and the other mothers who gathered mornings for coffee thought the various cars at my house indicated I was "taking in laundry." Probably this explains why neighbors no longer looked me in the face or spoke when we met.

I had to rethink my vow that, "Nobody is going to drive me out of my town." All this time the girls were free to visit their father and the elders whenever invited. When they returned to me, they were unmanageable and angry because they had been drilled, "Your mother does . . . and your mother does that . . . ." It came from all sides. Bill and the elders had only tolerated each other during our marriage. Now it appeared that they took turns investigating where I went, what I did and with whom. They even shared the information with each other. What a cozy arrangement! Before, I had been threatened with institutionalization. Now my every move was being watched and reported on, both to turn the children against me and/or to have me declared an unfit parent.

Putting my pride aside, I took my week's vacation and hired a housekeeper to watch the girls. This gave me an opportunity to investigate and evaluate other areas in the state for employment, education, and housing. After deciding on a city 225 miles away; I returned, submitted two-weeks' notice, packed up the whole caboodle and attempted to move.

Knowing the skullduggery that was going on, I made the mistake of I confiding my plans to mother. (Apparently, I still could not believe that a mother could double-cross her only child.) Within hours, I received court papers denying my right to remove the children from the area. After a talk with my lawyer and a chat with the judge, we three went on our way 225 miles north.

Thank goodness that the oil checks began to arrive because it took a couple of weeks to land a full-time stint at a furniture-manufacturing firm. I came with glowing references from recent employment and the manufacturers' representatives. The new job was to update the records of the firm's national sales representatives. My mistake was not having a written contract. The clerk-typists figured if I could do it, they could also. Besides they had been there longer. So, to keep peace in the family—and because of a business slump after Christmas—I was considered expendable. Now I see it as another nudge.

Mother came to visit us (yes, this is the same mother, but I was on my own turf now) and check out the new apartment. She went with me for an interview at the Interlochen Arts Academy (IAA), a pre-professional secondary school. Bless her heart, it was her white hair (and probably her personality) as much as my references which charmed the financial wizard who interviewed me. Now I was employed, the girls were in school, and I had 200-plus miles of insulation. Life was good.

Moving from "my town" was a far more challenging trek into the unknown for the children, I knew. They would leave behind their father, the elders, their friends and their activities. Looking back, most of the incidents pointed toward getting "out of harm's way." The morning after we moved into our new quarters, five-hours' drive from the home town I had vowed not to leave, the mood-altering medication I had been taking was no longer necessary or helpful. It seemed reasonable to dispose of the remainder, which I did. The recent past had been a not-so-pleasant nudge to try new territory.

Fortunately, the girls soon began to make friends at their new schools. Cynthia continued her violin lessons with an excellent teacher who helped her attain a higher skill level. Her improved playing helped her win a summer scholarship to the National Music Camp (NMC). Winter came, bringing with it the promised, long, ice-skating season. The ice rink, located across the street in the same block, didn't close until lights out at 9 o'clock. For almost two months, Linda came home from school to get her skates, requested hot soup for a quick meal, and returned from the rink at lights out—a schedule she thoroughly enjoyed.

After leaving the furniture factory, I started work at NMC and its alter ego, in winter the IAA. Both entities were wonderful and interesting places to work. Both offered preprofessional training to students in music, art, dance, and academics. Although I started working in IAA student accounts, I moved to Personnel, Purchasing and finally into IAA student recruitment.

Cynthia had always understood that if she wanted a college education, she had to excel. She was a diligent student in academic as well as violin studies. She woke herself early to study during the quiet time before the rest of us got up. Her rewards were scholarships in both areas.

Linda, now 12, started dance lessons and continued ice skating. Both girls had studied piano before leaving the home town, so both could read music and knew the piano keyboard. (Their piano teacher was able to seat the sisters on a piano bench, without fighting, long enough to play a duet or two.) But Linda was more the high-energy type, sometimes reminiscent of the old saying, "like a fly on a hot griddle." She did well with dance, far better than piano—and even performed in an outdoor ice-skating show which required hours of outdoor practice while temperatures were in the teens.

The following summer, we rented a cottage located near the NMC campus, near the lake and within easy walking distance of where I worked. The girls kept busy with NMC classes during the day. Cynthia continued in a small, four-piece-string-instrument class. Linda took dance lessons and made herself spending money by baby sitting. Evenings the three of us attended one of the many music or dance activities nearby in the Camp.

One rainy day, while I was working and the girls didn't have classes, Linda decided to bake brownies. Cynthia was sitting on the porch reading when she heard Linda puffing and fuming. That noise came from the kitchen. It was Linda removing the brownies from the oven. What Cynthia saw when she came to investigate was her sister holding a pan of brownies faced by an angry-looking rattlesnake. Cynthia picked up a nearby shovel and killed the snake. To this day we sometimes remember "the day the snake came to eat Linda's brownies."

It was a busy, wonderful, fun-filled summer. Even as I reveled in the times we had together, I often had this niggling thought that all too soon, the girls would be going their own ways. And how could I bridge the separation when they left?

At the end of summer camp over Labor Day weekend, we moved back into our apartment in town. Now that the girls had separate areas of expertise, they seemed more at ease in each other's company. Growing up as an only child,

I had no background in family rivalries or politics. I always thought the continuous conflict between them was the sibling rivalry I had read about—something to be expected and gone through. But now the girls tell me they "used to hate each other." Whatever it was, their mutual tolerance increased as they applied themselves to their separate areas of interest.

For me, continued study led to doing more frequent solo work in various churches and becoming a paid soloist in the summer. (Being paid for singing is usually a sign to others that one is successful—but it is far more important to the self that one has achieved a dream.)

This Labor Day weekend was significant in many ways—not just that the Beetles' movie was playing at the local theater, although that was involved. The important aspect was that, while working in the personnel office, I had filed applications received for the vacant English Department chair position. After scanning one application, I thought to myself, "He looks like a keeper. I wonder if he has a sense of humor." That was when photos were part of the application process and this photo showed a distinctive, Lincolnesque chin. The chin and the lines in the face made me wonder about a sense of humor. I soon discovered not only did he possess humor, but he also had all the qualities I valued. "He" had a name—Ralph,

He had visited campus for the successful job interview the preceding spring. When he checked in as a new faculty member in the fall, I invited him and other school faculty members for a Labor Day afternoon get-together. He arrived with some refreshment; the others neither showed up nor called. Cynthia and Linda had gone to see the Beetles' movie. Midway through the afternoon, they called to ask if they could stay to see the movie through again. He didn't seem to mind being the only guest. We spent the time until the movie was finished getting better acquainted.

That fall when school began, Cynthia, now a senior, was identified as a National Merit Scholar. She had spent the summer at NMC as the winner of the violin scholarship. It came as no surprise that she was accepted at IAA that fall. A few days later, as an excited Cynthia was transferring her belongings from our car to the school dormitory, my new friend, Ralph, and I crossed paths, I lamented, "I don't know how to deal with crossing this bridge."

Ralph answered, "And it's right now!" He understood well what I meant. We had been discussing the bridge-crossing earlier.

Right away I discovered it would be unwise to leave Linda alone in the apartment where the three of us had lived. The apartment was located 20 miles from where I worked. Before Cynthia checked into the IAA dormitory, the two girls had been company for one another when I had to be absent. However, now Linda had to spend time alone before and after school when I was at work.

Fortunately, a house near the campus was available. It was within walking distance of work. Also, the bus to Linda's school in town picked up other local students who were not enrolled in IAA. Perhaps Linda was not in actual physical danger alone in our apartment in town, but neither had she the protection of an older person. The great advantage of the house near campus was that the three of us could be together more often than if home base were in the city.

Ralph and I began seeing more of each other. While he was helping us move from the city to our new location, Linda and Ralph became friends. When she tried to address him but couldn't remember his last name, he suggested, "Just call me Sam." From then on within the family, Ralph has been "Sam."

After that, Linda became quite fond of Sam. In fact, when she found out his birthday was late in October, she wanted to bake him a birthday cake. I agreed that it was a fine idea if she could get his approval. After he accepted, she tried the oven in the recently-rented house. It didn't work. Sam said she could use the stove in his cabin on campus. So, with his permission, she cleaned his stove and then baked the cake. It was a work of art. The party was a success and no snake came to spoil her culinary achievement plus Sam was pleased to have his stove cleaned.

During Christmas vacation, the four of us visited the elders. After introducing Ralph to mother, I took the laundry to the laundromat—we needed clean clothes and my absence afforded mother and Ralph a chance to get better acquainted. Ralph soon appeared at the laundromat visibly upset. True to her colors, mother had given him her spiel on "Jeane's poor choice in men." He withheld comment but avoided any unnecessary conversation with her.

School resumed for everyone after Christmas vacation. In addition to being Head of the English Department at IAA, Ralph also taught skiing and horseback riding to students. On one of his days off, when he was not doing either of the latter, I asked if he thought I could ski. Two or three years previously, I had had surgery on the right knee for torn meniscus cartilage after which the surgeon had warned, "No twisting motion." Twisting was The Dance at the time, but I neither danced it nor wished to. But I never related twisting to skiing. One weekend we borrowed ski boots for me from Ralph's friends and headed toward Boyne Mountain where the Olympic ski hopefuls often practiced.

We had chosen a warm, sunny day which followed deep snow and piercing cold. These changes had made the surface snow crisp, icy, and slippery. I was proud to have used the tow rope getting up the Bunny Slope twice, but the last time I fell coming down. Ralph asked if he could help me up. I declined but asked him to lift the ski off my leg. He realized there wasn't any ski there to lift! After brief examination, he decided I had broken that right leg—did I twist it? I don't know. Because there was no ski patrol or first aid on the Bunny Slope, it took a while to get me to the local clinic.

The bad news from the clinic x-ray was I had broken both bones in the lower leg, one high and one low. The good news was that the clinic could not reduce the breaks with a pillow splint and they were not equipped to do the necessary surgery. It would have to be performed elsewhere—hopefully nearer home.

In the choice between surgery at the local hospital and going back to town near my children (and Ralph's work), I opted in favor of nearness to family. We called the orthopedic surgeon who had performed the previous knee surgery. He said he would wait at the hospital for us. This he did.

After viewing the x-rays, he pronounced, "Well, you'll never walk again," and waited expectantly. (He always gave the worst scenario first.)

"What do we do now?" I inquired.

"We can operate tomorrow. You'll be in the hospital for a year," was the reply.

"Then let's operate tomorrow. Now may I have something to eat. I haven't eaten since early breakfast?" Earlier I had been advised not to eat in case surgery was imminent. But now it was close to 8:30 in the evening. The doctor nodded consent. I tried unsuccessfully to eat the salad, the only food the nurse could find. Ralph offered to help feed me because the sleep medication had already made me too drowsy to manage a fork; but I refused.

When I awoke the next day, my right leg was encased in a still-damp cast from above the toes to my upper thigh. Only the heel and the toes protruded. For the next two days (and nights), every time a nurse came by me, she felt my toes.

Ralph jokingly remarked, "Maybe they (the nurses) have a 'thing' for toes." But they felt the toes to check for warmth; coldness would have indicated loss of circulation.

A few days later, when the doctor discharged me to go home, he ordered no walking or weight on the right leg with its full-length, 25-pound cast. I went home with a crutch for the left arm (the right shoulder was too weak to support a crutch). In answer to my question about how to get up and down necessary stairs, the doctor's terse reply was to wear slacks and scoot on my fanny. Once home, I was able to get from the car seat to the stairs and scoot up the stairs. However, with the full-length cast and only one, not-so-strong arm, I couldn't pull myself up to stand. I flailed and wailed. But the cast was heavy; it didn't bend; and I was forced to ask for help. Although my independence was threatened, there was no alternative. Ralph was willing, but he was wise enough to wait for a request. In fact, he had already anticipated my predicament by renting a portable wheelchair.

Very soon, my boss, the Academy office manager, came to visit. The purpose of her visit was not offer assistance or to express concern. It was to tell me that they wouldn't hold my job for me. My reply, without consulting the doctor, was that I would return to work the next Monday—about four days away.

Linda returned home from the faculty family Ralph had arranged for her to stay with during the few days I was gone. She was able to help me before and after school. In the morning, Ralph came to get me and the wheelchair and took us to work. After work he brought me home. He saw to it that we had everything we needed from town and Linda was able to walk the short distance to the local grocery. In short, Ralph was my steady, dependable, loyal friend all through the three months until the cast came off. Thanks to his support, I didn't lose my job although I felt that possibility snapping at my heels. I knew my job thoroughly and did it well; but I was aware that I had crossed someone higher on the ladder. For now, I was safe.

Knowing, now, that the world would not rock if I asked Ralph for help, I mentioned the difficulty in taking a bath. A "spit" bath at the sink just didn't fill the bill. So my trusty friend came up with two excellent suggestions. First, he brought some "turkey bags"—large, plastic bags which I could pull over the plaster cast and secure around the upper thigh, above the cast, with rubber bands and a paper clip.

Then he showed me how to take one of my wooden, kitchen chairs; place it with two legs in the tub and two legs on the bathroom floor; sit in the chair and swing my legs over the edge into the tub. I could remain sitting on the chair or standing up (if I was brave and foolish) to take a satisfying shower. I could exit the shower by reversing the procedure. This worked well until the cast was removed.

The cast came off three months later when the x-rays showed that the bones had knit properly, I reveled in the freedom of walking and, apparently, my strength had returned.

At the end of the academic year, Cynthia graduated from IAA class of 1965 with honors. She was accepted with a scholarship at the college of her choice. She wanted to invite her classmates to a graduation party. It was easy for them to attend a celebration at our house because we lived so close to campus. She described the kind of party she wanted to be like a stand-up, cocktail party but without alcoholic beverages.

The night before the event we prepared for the party. The guests arrived, but the honoree was a little late. Her father had come to attend graduation, taken her for a ride, but he didn't bring her back on time. Mother, true to form, was "insulted" and threw a fit because we had prepared the party elements the night before without consulting her or asking for her assistance.

After the party, the elders went down the road a bit to the one-and-only bar (which was affectionately known by faculty and staff as "Northern Campus Limits.") When they finally joined us for supper, mother worked herself up to a frenzy shouting that she had been badly treated and insulted and they would go home right then! I tried to reason with my stepfather because a 225-mile drive, starting after 5 p.m. and several hours of drinking, was dangerous. He smiled meekly and said, "What else can I do?" So, off they went. Thank goodness they made it safely.

In a short time, Cynthia was due to start work during the summer at a religious school about twenty miles distant. Linda was still baby sitting for campus faculty and Ralph was moving out of his housing according to the terms of his contract. Most of the faculty at IAA (like Ralph) vacated their premises which were then allocated to the summer NMC faculty and staff. He planned to return to his sister's in Ohio. We were very close—as the tabloids would say, "an item." Cynthia had not realized we were so close.

Because the school was out in the country and there weren't alternative eateries, faculty and staff (like me) often ate with students at noon. And sometimes the three of us (Ralph, Cynthia and I) ate at the same table. If Ralph and I were planning to do something together, I would mention my date was, "Sam;" because "Sam" he had become to the family. The question of identity was solved because there was only one other Ralph on the campus—the skunk the students had named "Ralph."

But it, "The Item" concerning Ralph and me, was conveyed through the woman who ran the school bookstore, whom the students called "Minnie the Mouth." Minnie learned it from the campus housekeeping maids. The same maid who cleaned once a week for Ralph also cleaned for me after I broke my leg. This is a perfect example of the Campus round robin.

We were married in July 18, 1965, after Ralph returned from visiting in Ohio. My beloved music teacher invited us to use her magnificent home located on the Peninsula overlooking Grand Traverse Bay for the wedding. Two dozen friends and faculty members surrounded us as we peered through the 75-pane glass window at the Bay sparkling below while we took our vows.

Our hostess—also the matron of honor—had surprised us with, "You're welcome to serve some bubbly." This meant we could offer a toast. That she, a Christian Science practitioner would permit, even suggest, an alcoholic beverage was very touching. However, we were even more astonished when she produced two-dozen. stemmed, crystal champagne glasses from her china cabinet. It wasn't until the last guests were arriving we discovered our hostess had no bottle opener. Cynthia took Linda and the car into town to get the bottle opener which would facilitate the ceremonial toast.

Our housing (part of Ralph's fall teaching contract) wouldn't be available until early September. The first six weeks after our wedding we lived in the house near campus and held a continuous yard sale to downsize the amount of furniture we had between us. Housing was a charming, furnished, two-bedroom duplex on campus. Between us we had more than enough to furnish a house. Some of it was used in the furnished apartment (housekeeping obligingly removed and stored some of the furnishings). Some of ours was stored in the basement of another, generous, faculty member for our future use. The remainder went into the yard sale. Some of my "treasures" were difficult to part with, but I've lived happily without them.

One of my most precious memories of all time concerns Ralph immediately mortgaging his beloved new auto, his Karman Ghia, to pay Cynthia's college costs. Aware that costs would run above the scholarship, I had assumed payments could be made on a monthly basis which would be covered by the oil checks. Not so. The college wanted costs prepaid, up front. His action ranks first place as a token of love and support from a brand-new stepfather.

At the beginning of the fall term, Ralph and I moved into our furnished duplex, Cynthia started her four-year stint at the college of her choice in Kalamazoo; Linda, a 9th grader majoring in dance, now was eligible to be enrolled as an IAA student living in the dorm because she was part of an IAA faculty family. The bridge I had dreaded crossing—separating from my children—was well under construction.

Occasionally, Linda joined our table with other students at lunch. And sometimes she took a short walk to our duplex during free time to make herself a peanut butter sandwich. The head of the dance department pointed out to her that nobody is willing to pay $25 a ticket to see a 200-pound ballerina. That didn't deter Linda. We just ceased having peanut butter in the house.

Perhaps it was because I had my brought my own, new-to-offices, IBM electric typewriter to work (the machine which made me equal to the able-bodied typists) or perhaps because I had done an outstanding job of enrolling incoming students, the cloud which had been hanging over me suddenly let loose. One morning without warning, the personnel manager stalked over to my desk, told me I was no longer employed, and ordered me to leave immediately. One look at his red, contorted face and I left. I had never worked so hard nor been so shamed and embarrassed before co-workers. I had never before been fired from any job.

I shed more than a few tears and experienced deep anger. Those feelings were aggravated when campus security was sent to my apartment demanding that I surrender my badge and uniforms. Certainly, I had no use for them and fully intended to return them on my own. The fact that security was sent on such an errand was truly devastating. Now, I realize it was another one of those nudges to get me back on the track.

One of the employees of a local CPA firm who did work for the Academy knew my work. Possibly he was instrumental in my being offered the job as office manager in his firm. Because working with taxes was not my cup of tea, after the tax season reached its crest, I applied for a social-work-type position advertised at the local hospital. To my surprise, I joined a small unit devoted to helping patients transfer from hospital beds to homes or assisted living. My co-workers were wonderful to work with, I learned a lot, and I thoroughly enjoyed what I was doing. I enjoyed the work so much I really didn't want to leave. But Ralph's employment plans changed at the end of spring semester—the end of the IAA contract period.

During this first year of marriage, Ralph and I enrolled in some college classes. He, of course, already possessed the master's degree. I had only an associate of arts (A.A.) behind me. But when Ralph saw how avidly I pursued the courses, he kept encouraging me to continue and helped me to do so.

Ralph's theory about employment was that after two years, a teacher either had to upgrade his training ("retread" he called it) or else move into another position. He maintained in that amount of time students knew his methods and his jokes. Thus he applied for and was accepted as assistant to the president of a two-year-technical college in southwestern New York State. Linda, now a 10th grader, moved with us. Cynthia came to New York with us to spend her summer quarter which was really her college vacation. She returned to college in Michigan in the fall. But we four spent the summer together.

Ralph immediately was thrown into his administrative duties, I worked as a secretary in a former oil refinery refitted to be New York State's first, post-secondary vocational school. Linda enrolled in a sewing class where we hoped she would meet and make new friends over the summer.

That fall, Linda began attending local dance classes with noticeable lack of enthusiasm. While at the Academy, she was in dance classes daily at least two hours a day. Here she showed little interest and did almost no practice until she decided to enter her high school's talent show. One evening when I returned from work, I was delighted to see Ralph (a/k/a Sam) teaching Linda how to do bumps and grinds to Al Hirt's record of "Cotton Candy." She didn't win the contest, but she was now known by the student body. She certainly had friends and acquaintances after that performance.

Ralph was still encouraging me to pursue a degree so I left the job at the vocational school to start the spring semester at what was then Geneseo State College (now State

University of New York at Geneseo). In addition to taking a full schedule of courses, commuting took an hour each way. The snow drifts and chill of southwestern New York are at least as unpredictable and forbidding as northern Michigan.

The new, college-faculty housing where we lived was not well insulated; worse, it was difficult to heat. Also, using electric heat was extremely expensive. No matter how high the thermostat, we couldn't stay comfortably warm. After that first winter, we looked for alternatives of which there were few in the little town of Alfred. This forced us to look in the outlying area.

June found us inspecting three farm properties about seven miles from the college where Ralph worked. All three belonged to a former patriarch who had built each of his two daughters a home. These two homes were now on the market. To me, the most-appealing offering was a ten-room farmhouse on one acre of land. Although it hadn't been lived in year-round for thirty-nine years, it did it have promise. It also had a small (decrepit) shed, a 120-foot-deep well, one electric circuit, and an outhouse.

The circle drive also serviced a huge barn on the adjoining land. Mr. Kent, the owner, stored certified, seed potatoes in that big, temperature-and-humidity controlled barn. "Potatoes have to be fooled that it isn't yet spring; otherwise they sprout and I can't sell 'em for french fries," Mr. Kent explained.

Goldenrod paralleled the two-lane, crowned, gravel road. As we approached the front of the house (the better-looking side which still showed some remnants of aged paint), the girls' smiles became more like forced grins. Once inside, the hardwood floors didn't offset the peeling, drooping, old wallpaper; nor did the lovely, birdseye-maple antiques Mr. Kent used while supervising his potato-crop employees in the summer modify the effect. The pitcher pump presented the only evidence of kitchen area. Neither upstairs nor downstairs offered a bath or toilet and except for a small, pot-bellied stove in the so-called kitchen area, no heating system graced the premises .

This 1901 turn-of-the-century, sturdily-built house used timber supports with the bark still on in the basement. Our first house inspection accomplished two things: it made the girls truly enthusiastic about going back to Michigan for the summer and, more importantly, Ralph and Mr. Kent shook hands on the purchase of the house.

By late June, the girls had left to spend the summer in Michigan, Cynthia at college and Linda at the farm. They didn't get to appreciate the uniqueness of the house transaction where Mr. Kent's attorney represented both us, the buyers, and the owner, Mr. Kent. The transfer was accomplished with a minimum of fuss and feathers. Apparently, both parties were satisfied with the handling of the situation.

July first, the two of us celebrated by moving into the farm house where our auspicious address was:

Pingry Hill

Andover, New York.

The first three days in residence, Ralph heaved the basement debris of previous owners out of the basement window while I unpacked boxes and found places for our possessions. I also discovered the colony of bees that, long ago, had taken up residence in the wall of the upstairs, west bedroom. They weren't aggressive, but neither were they easily evicted. But that comes later.

On July 4th, Ralph left for a three-week, job-related conference 300 miles distant. In his absence, the contractors we had earlier signed agreements with started on their construction projects. These included insulating the house; creating a bathroom in the largest, upstairs bedroom; installing a sump pump; adding greater electrical service; and installing a leach bed to accommodate our sewer needs. In Ralph's absence, I answered questions according to my understanding of the ongoing work. The man constructing the leach bed asked me if I was sure we wanted a 750-gallon tank for the leach bed.

"Isn't that what you and Mr. Dille agreed upon? I countered.

"Yes, but how many people in your family? Do you have a dishwasher or washing machine?" he asked.

"There are three of us now and we don't have either a dishwasher or washer. Why do you ask?"

The contractor explained that if we had those appliances, we might need a larger leach bed to dispose of the waste water. And because there was thin topsoil over rock, he would have to blast in order to install a larger, 1000-gallon tank in the leach bed. After a phone conference with Ralph outlining the situation, we agreed to agree on the previous arrangement of 750-gallon size. To my relief, it was not necessary to blast.

One afternoon when I greeted the contractors as they were preparing to leave, I questioned whose black-and-white dog was hanging around. I was told that the dog had simply drifted by earlier and probably stayed because they fed him leftovers and offered him water. He was company during the evenings until Ralph returned. The dog barked at cars traveling the road a quarter of a mile away parallel to our road, but he didn't seem to chase anything close to the house. When Ralph beheld the dog, he described the animal as a border-collie mix who, we suspected, was near-sighted. Since the dog elected to stay after the contractors left, we gave him a name: "Alfredo" similar to Alfred, the small town nearby. Alfredo distinguished himself by catching prairie dogs which he left on the doorstep to be admired. If the carcass was moved, he would retrieve it and return it to the altar of the doorstep for another day or two of further admiration.

Early one morning, before the exterminators, the driver of the propane, heating-gas truck arrived and made ready to winch the tank onto its foundation west of the house.

Although this was mid-July, the air was still cool on the west side in the shade. As he was uncoiling the copper tubing which would connect the furnace with the outdoor tank, I spied a couple of bees buzzing overhead.

"You might want to come back in the evening when it's cool and the bees have hived," I suggested.

"Lady, I don't get overtime," he answered as he continued with the wire.

So, I left to go to class. When I returned that evening about 9:30, he was just finishing up the connection. The bees were quiet and nowhere to be seen. They were safely tucked into their wall space somewhere on the west side of the house.

In early September we were preparing for the possibility of early winter. We tried discouraging the bees with Raid and Black Flag. None of the suggested remedies was successful. Finally we had to call an exterminator who blew cyanide between the walls. The bees were not easily disturbed. Two applications were necessary. Each time we were advised to sleep on the opposite side of the house. Although we saw no more of the bees, their scent remained—especially on warm days. This reminded me of the words of a song, "The song is ended but the melody lingers on."

Still aimed at a degree, I continued to commute to Geneseo for a full schedule of summer courses and worked half days in the conference department of at the local college, Ralph's employer. I saw the contractors mornings and evenings of their working days. My routine was rather rustic or spartan. On the way home, I stopped in the village for food and ice which I kept in a plastic ice chest. (I'll bet that grocer thought I had a party every night when I picked up the ice.)

With the single electric outlet, I could heat water for coffee or to wash when I wasn't using the outlet to cook with the electric skillet. Each evening I had to remember to sweep up a 12-inch-round pile of dead bee bodies in the upstairs, west bedroom. The one time I forgot to empty the sweeper bag, I was roughly reminded that bees are "bodies." And their decaying scent lingered whenever I used the sweeper.

After he returned from the month-long conference, Ralph looked around the room where the kitchen ought to be and said, "This is ridiculous. Let's go to town." The next day our kitchen sported all the essentials including the stove of my dreams and a new refrigerator. Ralph built some additional working space. Then he measured the wall space. We picked out a provocative and expensive French print wallpaper. I didn't know he could wallpaper. Not only was he an expert wallpaperer, but he also transformed that area into a functional, pleasant, attractive place to cook.

An interesting event happened during the installation of the sump pump. The dependable water supply we would require from that 100-plus foot deep well wasn't going to happen using a pitcher pump. A sump pump was essential to bring the water up from such a depth. The pump man made the necessary connections and wired in the new, Red Jacket motor. But it wouldn't pump! He returned the motor to the hardware store and brought out another new, Red Jacket motor. This one didn't work either. When the third, new motor gave the same results, we stood in a circle around the pump: Ralph, the hardware store employee, the pump installer, the Red Jacket representative, an engineer friend from the college where Ralph worked, and I. We shook our heads in disappointment and disbelief.

The engineer friend said, "I don't know how to fix this pump, but I can get you water which will serve for the present." He went back to his lab at the college, returned with a motor and hooked it up to suck water from the cistern. This did work satisfactorily for the interim.

A few days later the pump man returned with yet another Red Jacket motor. He explained that the three, former motors (and who knows how many more?) had been wound backwards. This properly-wound, Red Jacket motor performed perfectly. Our friend, the engineer, installed the new pump with our grateful thanks.

We also purchased wallpaper for both upstairs and downstairs. In a rush to see improvement, we started papering the walls around the new, front door one late afternoon. By evening, the entire front room was completed. What a difference that made!

By the time Linda returned in September, her bedroom walls had been heavily-insulated, new wallboard applied, the walls papered and the woodwork painted. She was delighted to discover that she also had a small desk area and a closet built in which hadn't been there before.

She spent a lot of time in her room. Like many teenagers, her concept of a clean, tidy room did not match her parent's expectations, so we avoided her room as much as possible. Later Ralph found a sign to tack on her bedroom door which proclaimed: "Danger! Teenager lives here!"

Many changes had taken place by the first of September. From the standpoint of comfort, inside plumbing and circulating, hot-water heat rank high. The upstairs bath, once a bedroom, was bright and large—perhaps the largest room in the house. And the shower bath had white-tile walls which pictured a scene of swimming goldfish. Ralph could have done without the swimming goldfish, but that was the only size tile-wall covering available to the contractor at the time. In Ralph's absence, I "went for the gold." The decrepit, torn wallpaper had been replaced to give the inside a clean, sleek, bright appearance.

Probably the greatest improvement occurred when Ralph applied Sears yellow, one-coat, exterior paint which really made the house sparkle. The paint job required 29 gallons and that is a lot of paint for a one-coat job. Jokingly, we maintained that the exterior wood had lacked paint for so long that it sucked the lids off the paint cans.

Another change was that the coming fall, all three of us would be going to school. Ralph had promoted himself from his administrative position back to the classroom which he preferred. Linda would be attending Andover High School.

The biggest change occurred when I was offered a position teaching business at a nearby vocational school. How did this come about? A friend of mine, who was offered the position, had already accepted another job. She and I had much in common—both of us had been in military service and both of us had spent years in business. The big difference was that she already had her bachelor's degree and teaching certificate. I just had the associate degree plus another year of college. But when the principal read my credentials and interviewed me, he said, "I'm looking for someone between a top sergeant and a clown. And you seem to fill the bill."

For the first time in my life, I had a contract, made a decent wage and the Board accepted me without the degree or certificate; it was within their power to do so. Teaching was like a walk in the park. I was just passing along what I had learned in 29 years of business. My philosophy was to teach from the job out. Besides typing and office courtesy, it included a lot of language skills, job-interview practice, and the inauguration of that school's first cooperative work experience program. If it sounds like I loved it, that's the way it was. Another aspect which sweetened the experience came from greater earning power. Added income made the house restoration proceed more rapidly.

How was this marvelous change to take place? How could I teach full time and continue classes? One night a week I took evening classes from 4 pm to 10 pm. And yes, I still commuted to Geneseo. With evening classes and summer school, I remained with the degree program.

Caught up in the move and the projects needed to make the house habitable for the winter, I hadn't investigated the Andover High school programs. It was my own fault that I was taken by surprise. But shortly before school opened in the fall of 1967, Linda and I visited the guidance counselor. He outlined the school's various programs. In addition to the academic core, they included vocational subjects such as business, licensed practical nursing, cosmetology, engineering drawing, auto repair and appliance repair.

When the counselor asked her choice, Linda sent me a challenging glance and replied, "Cosmetology." At sixteen, she was old enough to choose. Without missing a beat I asked her if she was sure this was what she wanted. Cosmetology was her choice. She obviously enjoyed it and completed the two-year sequence. Although she never passed the state board license exam, the background she acquired in biology and chemistry came in handy for the ten years she managed a cosmetics department in a Wal-Mart store.

During the school year, I taught business classes from 9 a.m. until 3 p.m. Monday through Friday at the Hornell, New York Campus of the Board of Cooperative Educational Services (BOCES), commuted one evening a week for class work at Geneseo, and continued with summer school.

The year 1969 was a vintage year. In June, Linda graduated from high school; Cynthia and I both received our bachelor's degrees. My degree wasn't in social work; it was a Bachelor of Science (B.S.) in sociology/anthropology, the program nearest to social work that Geneseo offered. Mine was the extreme pleasure of attending Cynthia's graduation ceremony. There I met the fellow she would later marry. But that was not the last of the surprises in 1969.

Ralph was so proud of me for completing the (B.S.) degree in 1969 at Geneseo that he showered me with gifts. One was a two-piece set of green luggage complete with a travel alarm. The other was a silver-like-metal reproduction of my diploma mounted on a walnut base ready to hang on the wall. He remarked, "Anybody who took 29 years to complete a degree should have more than a piece of paper to show for it." His gift hangs on my "ego wall" nearby in my work room.

About ten days after Linda graduated from high school, she announced that she and her boyfriend planned to wed immediately. He had just returned from a third tour in Vietnam. As soon as they were married, he would return to Oklahoma so he could finish out his last three months of duty. The plan was that she would wait for him here at home.

Just how this marriage was going to be accomplished was right up there in the miracle category because the State of New York required a ten-day waiting period after the license was issued. There were only six days before he had to leave to return to Oklahoma. The details of now this wedding could be arranged were still to be discovered.

Her timing was brilliant. Guests were already arriving as she told us this, so we put discussion on hold. After they left, we could ask questions like, "Where," "when," and "how." Dinner was a blur and evidently conversation wasn't too spicy. Guests later said they had enjoyed the food and the conversation. And although they were dear friends, we longed for them to disappear so we could clear the deck and get some answers.

Linda was an attractive, social being who had dated lots of fellows. But Dennis, the groom-to-be, was easy to know and easier to like. He also seemed to have more maturity and more to offer than any other of her friends. My private opinion was that she was more in the marrying mood than he. But this shows how wrong a mother can be. Apparently he was as enthusiastic as Linda.

When the guests had gone, Linda revealed that the couple had been to see our family doctor for required blood tests that afternoon. He was a good and true friend of ours who asked if she had told her parents about their wedding plans. When she replied to the contrary, Linda was afraid the doctor would tell us first, so she hurried home to break the news.

Now to the wedding plans.

I asked, "Do you want to be married at home?"

"No," she replied.

"In church?"

"No."

"Well, just how are you going to accomplish this wedding?" was my last question.

"By a Justice of the Peace," she countered.

At midnight we agreed that nothing much could be accomplished over the weekend. Dennis, our son-in-law to be, departed. Linda went to bed. I looked forward to Monday morning when I might be able to ask a friend for information and perhaps for assistance.

My friend, Kathryn, was the wife of the local Justice of the Peace; but Linda didn't know that. Kathryn suggested she and I meet to chat with her husband who might have some "possibilities" we hadn't thought of. He did, indeed, seem sympathetic and asked that the couple visit him in his office.

The Justice of the Peace turned out to have a wealth of information and certain powers too. After listening to the facts—that the groom was returning from a third span of duty in Vietnam and that his ten-day leave ended shortly—this kind man made the proper arrangements to amend the waiting period. The couple was married two days later (in church with my friend, Rev. Wolters presiding).

For a long time—years—I had been dreading the time when both of the girls would be gone. But the night before the wedding, I didn't see any sign of packing. So, I asked, "Aren't you getting ready for the trip to Oklahoma?"

She surprised me with, "No. Dennis wants me to go, but I didn't think you would let me. So I'm going to stay here with you until he gets discharged."

With surprise and disbelief, I went downstairs to talk it over with Ralph. "I don't think it's right for Linda to enjoy the status of marriage but not assume the responsibilities. And people do gossip. That's not fair to Dennis." I discussed with Ralph my reservations.

Ralph suggested trying to reason with Linda—to make her see how lonely Dennis would be without her. I also pointed out how lonely she would be as a married woman who wouldn't be dating or hanging out with unmarried friends and what devastating gossips she knew the locals could be.

"Sam and I think you should go with Dennis. He would be very lonely without you," was difficult to say because I really dreaded seeing her go.

"Dennis wanted me to go, but I didn't think you would let me," she replied.

"We certainly think you should go. In fact, Sam said that if you didn't go, he'd pack your suitcase, put it on the front porch, and lock the door," was my parting shot.

At this, Linda grinned with pleasure, pulled out her suitcase and began piling clothes on the bed. She was doing what she wanted and I was losing my younger daughter. Not really "losing," but our roles would never be quite the same. Although what I had always wanted was to see the girls become independent women who chose their own ways and who possessed the strength to face the risks of their own decisions, I felt a terrible dread. Marriage is a high-risk decision and no one can tell what the outcome will be. Legally and chronologically she was old enough to marry. The maturity, if it wasn't already there, should surely follow.

We had been hoping she would at least have a marketable skill when she left school and home. However, one failed try at the state Board of Cosmetology exam was followed by a snowstorm which prohibited our driving her to the next exam site, Rochester, 70 miles way. And after the wedding bells rang, there was no regard for taking tests. Marriage filled her life.

Now both girls were settled in their new lives away from home. Cynthia was working for the telephone company near her birthplace in Michigan but 500 miles away from us. And Linda had her own place in Wellsville not too far distant in space but the ease and comfort of visiting in-laws was not well established. The ten-room, farm house was much quieter since we no longer had a student in school.

When the heavy snowstorms came that fall, we were reminded that we were no longer on the school-bus route. Forget the promise of postal service delivery. The snow plows simply plowed around us. Actually we were not too surprised because the road maintenance crews had earlier demonstrated some strange customs. In summer or good weather, the huge road-maintenance truck/plow often sped by on the gravel road at 40 mph with the plow blade raised high above the road surface. This action conveyed the loud message, "We're thirsty." Either our only neighbor—a quarter-mile distant—or we would hang something on the mailbox—a six-pack or a pint—to assuage their thirst. With no student at home for the school bus, that winter (1969) we were snowed in for two weeks; the subsequent and last winter (1970), we were snowed in for ten days.

Luckily, we had kept on hand enough food and fuel for an emergency. Without television, all that uninterrupted time permitted me to knit all my yarn, sew all the fabric, rearrange the books and file all papers and music. At one time, we had 13 feet of snow in and around the road to our house before the equipment of two townships plowed us out.

In June 1969, with the B.S. degree in English behind me, I finished closing up my business classroom for the summer. That same summer I started work on the master's degree. For the next two years, I taught full time and took evening classes and summer school to finish up the required master's of science (M.S.) program at Geneseo.

At the same time, Ralph was saying, "I need the terminal degree." He had waited until Cynthia and I had our bachelor's degrees, Linda had finished high school and married. Now it was his turn. He applied to the five schools which offered the degree he needed. He chose Ball State University (BSU) in Muncie, Indiana because it offered both acceptance into the English doctoral program and a fellowship. No way could I see myself remaining in New York, maintaining this beautiful house and fighting the snow in the winter. A better alternative was to go to Indiana and attend BSU with him.

A few weeks into that last New York summer school, Ralph insisted I remain on Geneseo campus during the week and return to our Pingry Hill home on weekends. He could see that I was becoming exhausted. The last required classes for my degree program were Organic Chemistry and Inorganic Chemistry offered in one, 12-week summer session. Although I gave it my best shot and all my waking hours, I barely passed. But I did pass and that was the important fact.

While I was at summer school, he was packing out the house on Pingry Hill which we had put on the market. All went according to plan: Ralph found us an apartment in Muncie, shipped what we needed and stored the rest. At the time my final exams were scheduled, he was in Muncie awaiting my arrival after I completed writing the final exam—the last hurdle. That's when the plan broke down.

In this pie-shaped, 300-seat conference room filled with hopeful Geneseo test takers, one of the deans was calling off the names of individuals to come forward and pick up their test packets. When he came to my name, he said in an ominous voice, "Dean so-and-so wants to see you right after the exam." All kinds of disturbing ideas troubled me. "Was Ralph all right? Had something happened to the children? Had there been an accident?" I did my best under the circumstances, but I was uncomfortably aware that I had not done well.

I headed for the administration building Immediately after finishing the exam. As I recall, I was able to speak with the Assistant to the President. Brushing away my tears (and being furious with myself for crying), I explained what had happened. He was kind, sympathetic, and he promised to look into the situation. This was some consolation, but it did not assure me that I would have the required masters-in-hand on which the job at BSU depended. Writing an acceptable exam was the last hurdle impeding possession of the degree. There was nothing else I could do to mend the situation.

By 3:30 p.m., I had transferred my already-packed belongings from the rented room into my car and departed for Indiana. I stopped about midway for a sandwich even though I wasn't hungry. In Muncie some 12 hours later, I found the motel where Ralph was staying. I could see his parked car so I knew he was there. But I didn't know what room he was in. Cold, tired out and frustrated, I found an all-night restaurant with a pay phone. After I dialed, the motel office phone must have rung for about ten minutes.

When the desk clerk finally answered the phone, he was understandably upset because it was almost 4 a.m. When I asked him to ring my husband, he declined saying the guests were asleep. I explained that I was the wife who had driven all night from New York, I was tired, I was cold, and I needed to talk to my husband. Finally, to my relief, I heard my husband's voice welcoming me and telling me his room number.

The next day we inspected and moved into our new quarters. Each apartment had one designated parking spot in front of it. The extra cars were parked down at the end of the street, behind the Church of God playground. On Sunday, after I unpacked my car and parked it in the "overflow parking" area, a group of teenagers was playing ball on the playground. I came back to the apartment commenting that I felt so safe with my car parked next to the Kingdom of God. Possibly I had mocked The Deity because the next morning I discovered that the front windshield of my beloved Volkswagen had been splintered—probably by a fly ball or a home run.

That December, I was permitted to re-take the master's exam in Muncie on the BSU campus. It was an informal arrangement. I sat on a bench next to the secretary of the the Chairman of the English Department writing on my lap. The exam evaluations came back from New York a few days later. The short message was that I had passed. One of the readers had commented that it was a darned good job. Now, at the beginning of the spring semester, with the master's degree in hand, I was eligible to join the other English doctoral students.

Our apartment was designed with two bedrooms upstairs. The second bedroom—the one with twin beds—was used mainly as an office. Although my electric typewriter dominated the room, each of us had a designated twin bed where we arranged our papers. None of the papers was filed, moved, or destroyed until assignments were fulfilled, the work complete and the grade received. Ralph preferred to use his manual keyboard in another area. He once described the operation as, "Jeane conducts from the console of her IBM. I hold forth on the keyboard of my manual Hermes downstairs."

Although our approaches differed, we respected and solicited the other's opinions. When the pressure was on to produce papers, we fell into a routine where we wrote for a couple of hours, then we gathered in the kitchen. Over a cup of coffee we discussed the progress we were making or the problems to be solved. Sometimes we'd read a sentence or a paragraph for the other's reaction. We used one another as sounding boards. I'm convinced that our writing became stronger as we shared ideas in a complementary way.

Sometimes we celebrated a special accomplishment by going to our favorite restaurant—the Carriage House. We considered making a deadline, finishing a paper or doing well on an exam worthy of rewarding ourselves. In fact, our celebrations were sufficiently frequent that the waitresses recognized us. They knew our preferences so well that often they could predict our orders.

One unique special (which wasn't on the menu) that the Carriage House offered to its "regulars" was a special showing of 1940s musicals on Saturday nights after the bar and restaurant were closed. The owners loved these musicals and evidently there was a ready audience for these movies. Nothing else kept us up until 2 a.m. Sunday mornings.

When we first moved from the higher altitude and lower temperatures of New York to the higher humidity and higher temperatures of Muncie, Indiana at the end of June 1970, summer came as a jolt. The following year, Indiana spring eased us into the more tropical climate. We learned to appreciate the advantage of air-conditioned autos and that life was about constantly traveling from one air-conditioned building to another. We also learned in Indiana that rain and snow fell horizontally and that when the wind blew from the direction of the Marhoffer meat-packing plant, the odor was the perfume of money to the employees and residents, but its fragrance was less agreeable to outsiders.

Toward the end of our first academic year in the program, we faced the question of economics. We had profited little from the sale of our New York farmhouse. That and the stipends from our fellowships and the student loans we had taken on were not sufficient to permit both of us to continue in the program. Luckily, the doctoral program was diversified so one could select specialties.

After getting a snootfull of what teaching the literature of the old bards was all about and the politics of administration, I veered toward linguistics—the study of language. This change boiled down to regrouping the work I had put into the English doctoral program so that I could emerge with a second masters—an M.A. in linguistics. My continuing in a teaching career did not require a doctorate. But I could certainly use the additional knowledge I would gain from a masters in linguistics. Therefore it seemed a good choice.

It all came down to the fact that Ralph, with his extensive teaching and administrative experience, needed the terminal degree. That degree was essential to progress in his chosen field. To me, the cutting edge was teaching business-related subjects to students who were ready to hit the job market. When we checked the requirements against my dossier, we discovered that with one more linguistics course after leaving BSU and with the completion of an acceptable research paper, I would have fulfilled the requirements for the master's degree in linguistics. This would be a second master's—this time an M.A. (Master of Arts). As frosting on the cake, I received the official notification that I had been accepted as a doctoral candidate at BSU—just to show everybody that I wasn't a quitter and hadn't been kicked out!

Unofficially, I received assurance that my former job in New York would be open in the fall should I return. There I would earn enough to live on and also supplement Ralph's income so he could complete his studies on campus at BSU. Neither of us was thrilled that, come September, we would be separated for a year. But this seemed a tolerable solution and a reasonable amount of time.

About this same time, the end of spring quarter, daughter Cynthia announced that she had set her wedding date for September 1. Knowing that he would not require as much living space—and in the effort to reduce overhead—Ralph applied for smaller, one-bedroom housing on campus at BSU.

We offered the engaged couple our second-bedroom furniture if they would come to get it. They borrowed a suitable vehicle one weekend and drove from Lansing, Michigan to Muncie to view and accept the furniture. Said they had seen an apartment but hesitated to rent it because they had no furniture. Now that they had the essentials, they could proceed with the apartment. Our space was now so limited that three mattresses from the outgoing furniture were piled on the bed where Cynthia slept. She said she felt like the Princess and the Pea sleeping on three mattresses.

After the wedding, Ralph returned to BSU and I had a small, furnished apartment in Andover, NY. Living in an apartment in a small town again was pleasant except for missing Ralph. Didn't miss the deep snow drifts of nearby

Pingry Hill, though. My neighbors were pleasant, friends at work included me in their activities, and the Christian Science Church in town hired me as their vocal soloist. The telephone company was delighted with our long-distance call activity.

Ralph drove from BSU to New York so we could spend some of Christmas vacation together. At spring break, when he joined me, we found a wonderful, old, deserted farmhouse that seduced us with its gorgeous, wood, living-room walls and giant, stone fireplace. Through friends I taught with, we were able to contact the owner and arrange to rent the place. In one short week, Ralph drove back to Muncie, packed up our belongings into a U-Haul Truck, drove the truck back to New York through a terrible snowstorm, and in we moved. At the end of the week, he took the bus back to BSU to finish out his school year. That's stamina.

Midway through summer, New York weather produced one of its heavy storms which caught us in the flood of June 1972. On our perch halfway up Bailey hill, we were safely above the flood waters which covered much of Steuben County. From our position of safety, we felt somewhat guilty that we couldn't offer shelter to some people whose homes were dangerously close to the rising water. But the roads to us were flooded. People in the lower areas could not have reached us.

With our well-stocked food pantry, we passed the time listening to flood reports and deciding whether to use Chlorox or boil water for ten minutes to make the water safe to drink. To our surprise, we discovered that the large, dilapidated building which was collapsing at the top of the hill was the former Carriage House from which Carriage House Road had gotten its name. Many of the locals came passing by, going uphill on Carriage House Road because the old timers remembered that road was the old throughway. Other roads might be flooded, but this one was always passable.

At the end of spring quarter, Ralph had completed his BSU course work. Except for the June flood, we enjoyed summer in the farmhouse on Bailey Hill. Although we loved the place, we remembered how quickly we could be so snowed in that we couldn't get to or from work. (We remembered all too well how easily one could become snowbound.) The good friend we had made who lived at the top of the hill offered to chauffeur us with his snowmobile when necessary. During heavy snows, he promised to meet us evenings at the bottom of our hill and taxi us to our residence, and the reverse if necessary in the mornings. But cell phones were not available then. Plus, we found the house had a complicated and difficult heating system to maintain in winter. Reluctantly, we had to say "no" to renting Bailey Hill for the following year.

Our former home, on Pingry Hill, was again on the market. During the previous winter, heavy snow had melted so rapidly that it filled the basement with water. No one had tried or been able to get the water pumped out in good season. Whether the structure was still secure no one could tell. Finally, in September, we opted to rent an apartment in one of the town's two apartment houses. This was our residence for the next three years.

The following summer, Ralph was part of a group of educators who spent a month visiting schools in Russia, Yugoslavia and Hungary. Because there was no way to communicate during his absence, we had made a plan for his return. I was to get a motel room near the Rochester airport where I would meet his returning plane late in the evening. By 5 o'clock, I was checked into the motel. His plane wasn't scheduled to arrive for another five hours. I passed the time by getting a snack and reading the paperback book I'd brought along.

By 9:30, I was waiting at the gate designated for his incoming flight from New York. Shortly after 10 o'clock, the plane—the only one arriving this late—started discharging passengers. Some rushed, others sauntered. But Ralph did not appear. By the time the flight crew emerged, it was apparent that no husband of mine would arrive. So I asked one of the attendants if all the passengers had deplaned. She replied to the affirmative. I asked her if the passenger list contained the name of my husband. After checking, she advised me that he was not scheduled on this plane. She suggested that I call the New York office to find out whether he was scheduled for the next plane. Because this was the last arrival of the evening, the airport was closing. There was nothing left for me except to return to the motel room.

Taking the attendant's advice, I called the airline in New York. The canned notice advised that the airline offices were closed until 7 o'clock the following morning. Next, although it was now 2 a.m. where she lived, I called my daughter, Cynthia, in Michigan because she had been listed on this trip as his next of kin. I explained that Ralph had not appeared and asked if she had heard from him. She now knew the motel's name and where I could be reached by telephone should he check in with her to find my whereabouts. At midnight I decided there wasn't much else to do except wait for the main New York airline telephone lines to open in the morning.

Out came the trusty paperback which was interesting enough to keep me from worrying until I fell asleep about 5 am. At 7 a.m., Cynthia called. She had already contacted the airline and Ralph was listed on the next departing plane which should arrive about noon. Only 13 hours later than I expected him.

When he arrived, he explained that his seat mate on the plane coming home was so talkative that he was not permitted to sleep. In fact, he hadn't been able to sleep for more than 36 hours. While he waited for his connecting flight at the New York airport, he fell so soundly asleep that airline staff was unable to awaken him. They transported him to a cot behind the scenes, put his wallet and passport under his pillow, and let him sleep until time to board his final flight the next morning. What a relief to see him after imagining him being retained in a Moscow hoosegow for some touristy infringement of local law.

The following year, both of us attended when a one-month program was offered through UNESCO (United Nations Educational Scientific and Educational Organization). This is the same agency which supported his previous summer's trip to Russia. We visited Hungary, Switzerland, Germany, France, and Denmark. Each country gave the background and philosophy of its educational system, provided visits to schools at all levels (I was the only one interested in and teaching vocational education—Ralph chose kindergarten and primary level although he taught at the community-college level). Hungary teachers taught us enough language so we could read menus or street signs, count, and other "necessary" terms.

Each country made certain that, with the assistance of outstanding, professional translators, we saw and enjoyed its major attractions. One lady had been trained to translate in six languages, but she had "just been assigned to master a seventh." We educators seldom had a language besides our own. Consequently, in Paris, we ate lots of fried potatoes because we recognized the word "pome" in "pome frits" on menus.

In France, our translator/guide showed us "a really proper castle" explaining that a "proper castle" was one with a moat. In Denmark, I tried in my rusty German to identify the bus to take us to the Viking Museum. I addressed my question to the riders of each of the seven buses. Finally, at the seventh bus, a lady with a British accent said, "If you spoke English, I probably could help you." We all laughed about that.

The post office in New York had accumulated a considerable amount of mail for us during our month-long absence. Before I had a chance to open it, I met my principal who asked if I had received a telephone call from Oregon. This piqued my curiosity so much that the first letter I opened welcomed me to a one-year, vocational-education program at Oregon State University (USO). I wondered how this happened.

Ralph recalled that earlier in the spring, my vocational supervisor had circulated a half-page memo listing six universities offering a year-long program. To be considered, one should enclose a biography and select the educational institution. As usual, by the time the memo filtered down to the trenches, the due date had expired. Knowing I was too late, I had tossed the form into the wastebasket.

But Ralph retrieved the wadded paper, smoothed it out and suggested all that was needed was to write a biography and to choose the school. We discussed the six schools listed. When I came to OSU, his comment was, "I've never been there." (Translation, "I find it interesting; I'd like to go there.") He also knew that I had loved the Seattle area ever since being stationed there during World War II.

Using the information on the letter of acceptance we had at hand, I contacted the head of this project at OSU. If he was surprised when I asked for information about the program, he didn't hesitate about giving a ten-minute description covering the program and the fellowship. My response was, "If I can get a year's leave of absence from my job, I'd be delighted to accept." The next day I met with the district superintendent who already knew more than I did about the program in question. He agreed to the leave of absence and sent me on my way with his good wishes.

Jubilantly, I returned home to convey my acceptance to OSU. I suddenly realized that I had created a whirlwind. The program was set to begin in less than three weeks. One of the first decisions was whether to take my 3-year-old Volkswagen, Ralph's newer Karman Ghia, or fly to Portland, Oregon and rent or buy a car to use while in the program. I decided on my Volkswagen, named "Arch." I liked and trusted Arch. He was very dependable. I felt that with Arch

I could drive up one side of a tree and drive down the other. He was superlative on mountains.

Checking the road Atlas, I planned to allow myself a week to drive the 2700 miles from New York to Corvallis, Oregon. But I couldn't persuade myself that I would actually be driving across the continent and living away from home for a year. Nor could I start packing the car. The day before I planned to leave, Ralph told me to put on the bed what I wanted and needed to take. Then he would load the car. Early on an August morning I was on my way to Corvallis.

I drove three days with the Atlas on the seat beside me, took Sunday off for rest, and arrived at my destination in Corvallis three days after my Sunday rest. Surprisingly, the further west I drove, the more courteous and pleasant were the people I encountered. At first, the waitpeople seemed to sling the food at customers. Smiles were more like grimaces because they didn't reach the eyes. When I reached Worthington, Minnesota, I noted a distinct change in people's attitudes. I almost reeled when the waitress greeted me with obvious friendliness and a smile that lit up her whole face. A friendly, "How about a cup of coffee?" was never more welcome.

So much of my travel found my little Volkswagen sandwiched between semis and impatient drivers of bigger cars. Many times overhead road signs were obscured by the height of over-the-road vehicles. Friendliness and quiet were a welcome respite between daily, 450-to 500-mile drives. The further west I drove, the more I became aware of this friendly, welcoming attitude.

I reached my destination during the lull when Oregon State classes were not in session and before actual project activities began. The timing was right to find the perfect apartment: only two short blocks from campus in a well-furnished fourplex with laundry facilities and my own parking spot. Unpacking the car took less than three hours. I made up the bed, checked the refrigerator and went looking for essential food stuffs, a few dishes and some eating tools. Then I dialed my New York home to let Ralph know where I was and that I had arrived safely. He immediately wired flowers to decorate my new digs.

Looking back on that trip, I realize this adventure really started shortly after Ralph and I married in 1965. Although I had learned to drive in a 1935 Ford with manual shift, I had driven only cars with automatic transmission since polio in 1952. In order to shift a manual transmission, I had to reach through the steering wheel D-ring with the left hand because I have no "push-away" with the right.

Pointing to his four-in-the-floor Karman Ghia, Ralph had said,"I think you can do it." So with that encouragement, I had taken the driver's seat, peered at the arrangement, and, as the British say, "Gave it a go" on the road past our apartment which had almost no traffic. Automatic shift had allowed me to ignore the joys and control of manual shift. But he had encouraged me to meet the challenge. What satisfaction and elation meeting the challenge gave me! Now, almost forty years later, I still thank the powers that be for allowing me to push my limits.

The vocational education program at Oregon State University (OSU) offered many options. During an early session with the project director, Dr. Joel Galloway, I heard the sentence, "If you come into the program with two masters, you can get a doctorate in a year." This caught my undivided attention because I had just received final thesis approval for my second masters from my committee at BSU. All that was left to complete the degree was to type it into its final form and submit the required copies. At this point, I quietly took aim for the doctorate in vocational education.

This group of eighteen "fellows" in OSU's program had been selected by state on a population basis, I was one of four who represented New York State. Further, I was one of two fellows who brought to the BSU vocational program two masters degrees. Maybe my lifetime goal of the Terminal

Degree moved from the "possible" into the "probable" zone. This next year promised a real challenge.

As the program swung into gear, for the first time BSU's English Department, computer-class requirement made sense. Three years earlier my knowledge of a computer's uses had been limited to documents. Heck, why fuss with computers when I could type documents on my IBM. The fact that a computer could file, add, analyze, reposition, and play with data simply hadn't percolated through. But when our class started learning how various statistical tools could be used to prove other functions; I was sold. In fact, several ideas appeared that would lend themselves to research. Through the class on statistics, I learned what tools might be used. And the fact that our fellowship program had built into it the charge or fee for use of the University's computer facilities made tantalizing daydreams.

The vocational training program, often combined with other activities in the Education Department at OSU, exposed us to education/teaching models with which many of us were not familiar. It also thrust us into exhilarating situations—such as the National Vocational Education Conference in New Orleans—where we participated and were swept up into new ways of thinking. New research, innovative vocational programs, professional contacts and recently-developed products broadened our interpretation of education. All of this reminded me of the old adage, "Knowledge is free! Bring your own container."

The structure of the fellowship led me through the steps of designing a research project formerly referred to as the "doctoral dissertation" now referred to as "thesis" or, slangily, "magnum opus." Through the machinations of statistical tools (and the University's computer), I settled on examining how important certain communication tasks were to mechanics (who certainly knew what they needed), employers and to seven levels of educators.

My contention had always been that the communication skills required by students headed for the job market had not been studied thoroughly. In fact, searching the Internet data base found no studies on the needs of job-entry-level mechanics. To find out exactly what job-entry-level skills mechanics need to be able to use, ask them. Nobody could answer those questions better than an entry-level, automotive mechanic.

My purpose was to determine the importance certain communication skills were to job-entry-level mechanics and how often they had to use them. Then compare how the mechanics agreed (or disagreed) with employers' and educators' evaluations. What did mechanics need that they hadn't been taught? When should that have been taught? Were their teachers remiss or had the teachers not been properly trained? The study was conducted through Lane Community College in Eugene, Oregon. Communication skills investigated were: verbal, handwriting, and composition skills.

All of this may sound complicated, but it really isn't. The computer used statistical analysis to see if mechanics, employers and educators agreed on what communication skills were needed. This analysis would tell how well employers and educators agree with what mechanics maintain is necessary.

The results of the study indicated that teachers of high school juniors and seniors were the only ones giving high priority to the required communication skills needed by workers. And, the further away the teaching level from job-entry workers, the less educators understood the kind and importance of industrial workers' communication skills.

These results paint a different picture from our education model of "scope and sequence" or "spiral" curriculum model where material is first introduced at the lower level. At the next level, the material is broadened and enhanced. Sequential levels are not merely rehashing previous studies;

they are continuously enriching and enlarging the concepts. Communication skills are, theoretically, introduced in elementary grades. From then on, it should pursue a continuous effort to "polish the product."

Ralph was able to get an unpaid leave from his teaching assignment in NY for the spring semester. He joined me at OSU before Christmas break and was on hand January 4, 1976 for my 52nd birthday and for the formal presentation of my research findings. Many members of the Vocational Education teaching staff, most of the fellow students, and one helpful friend from Lane Community College attended. Although the tradition is that attendance is by invitation, several surprises appeared when many of the uninvited, who had previously held themselves aloof, arrived. But I appreciated their support.

At the beginning of the program we had been introduced to numerous faculty members. These faculty were available to chair our thesis committees and to help us jump the hurdles. Their responsibility was to help us through writing and presenting the document. I chose an individual about my daughter's age. Later I found out that I was the first student he had been assigned to as committee chair. I chose him because he had already published two, well-received textbooks. The fact that he wrote and published these while a full-time faculty member convinced me he had the discipline of a writer and I trusted that he would make me jump the necessary hoops.

At our first meeting he asked, "Can you write?" To answer his question, I pulled out two papers written for previous courses. The design of one paper obviously interested him. I chose to elaborate on the one which interested him. He agreed to be my thesis advisor and suggested the use of further research on communication skills as the subject.

After I had officially presented my thesis (which meant I had jumped the last hurdle) my chairman gave his copy of the document to the dean of the department. In the next all-school faculty meeting, she held the document aloft and announced, "I want to see more work like this." Subsequently my chairman became assistant dean. I like to think that perhaps my chairman's first graduate student's research contributed to his promotion.

Two department members had written a grant for funds to investigate various vocational education projects funded by the State of Oregon. The project was designed to identify projects or programs which were successful and which had the potential for being replicated. Having established myself as a writer and researcher, I was invited—employed— to work on the project. Now I was an employee of OSU, part of the teaching staff. Also, I was involved in creating the design of the research. My experience in filing came in handy when locating the documents relevant to the project. The documentation was warehoused in the Oregon State Department of Education in Salem, Oregon.

The short title of the new project was "Promising Practices." Definition of just what comprised a promising practice was, was established with the help of the advisory committee. The committee established criteria for identifying projects which were "promising." Promising meant the projects could be replicated. Committee-selected criteria were: the projects must focus on students as the target; projects must identify the materials, people or accessories necessary to accomplish the goal; and projects must include a person or a document/manual to recreate the project.

These criteria determined what projects, located all over the State of Oregon and dealing with all levels of education, would be included. So, after sifting through the Department of Education's files, a list of those which seemed to fulfill the criteria was selected. This list was offered to the advisory committee and, together with project staff (including me as a staff member), the final list of projects which fitted the selection criteria was identified.

Visiting the programs—if they were still in progress—or contacting the people responsible for creating them—was followed by writing descriptive summaries of the program. These visits took staff members to all of the state areas and all levels of education. As one of the "visitors," I was now eligible to be addressed as "Dr. Dille," to sign out a state-owned vehicle (with required authorization), to visit the various locations and to enjoy many perks that being a faculty member and possessing "the terminal degree" accorded.

Ralph described getting the degree as jumping a bunch of hurdles. This was a very special hurdle. I had given it my best shot. Now I was enjoying some of the rewards.

Having Ralph with me to share these experiences made them more exquisitely rewarding. Often, he joined the group for meetings, workshops, or field trips. Among other activities, he took a class on media (which he called "The Toy Shop"). He worked his way through 42 projects which had been designed to enhance educational presentations.

At graduation time, he had the option of attending the ceremony in the crowded gymnasium or watching the doctoral students on closed-circuit TV walk across the stage, one by one, as they were "hooded" (when the dean puts the hood over your head and congratulates you). The TV picture is close-up and centered upon the individual. As the Dean put the hood over my head and settled it on my shoulders, I looked into his face and thought, "You look so much like my son-in-law."

All was not rosy. The morning of the ceremony Ralph took me aside to tell me that Cynthia had planned a surprise. She had arranged to fly from Michigan to Oregon so she could attend my graduation. But she had suffered a slight stroke which forced her to cancel those plans. The stroke took most of the sight of one eye but spared the rest of her body. As Plan B, she had set up a three-way conference call later in the day connecting herself, her sister, Linda, and ourselves in Oregon. Two of my goals were linked: my daughters and the doctorate.

With Ralph beside me, all Oregon adventures took on new luster. We ate Mo's chowder in Newport; we visited Tillamook (where my grandparents had spent the last 20 years of their lives) and went through the Tillamook Cheese factory; we visited Seattle which I had longed to return to after being stationed at Bainbridge Island during World War II. While in Seattle, we purchased the foot-high, wooden, Indian totem I had long wished for. It stands in our entryway.

He accompanied me to visit a promising-practices site at Paisley, Oregon—right in the middle of the state. In this high school, students were brought by their ranching families to sites where buses picked them up. The buses then carried students the remaining 60 miles to the school. After school, the buses returned the students 60 miles to where their families picked them up. Obviously education had a high priority to the entire family.

Students at Paisley School had been expecting us. Not only did they give us a warm welcome, but they had also designed the menu for the lunch we would share with them that day. They had selected their own favorites which included home-made cinnamon rolls. Because of icy traveling conditions, we arrived later than expected. However, not one student lined up for the usual, available, second helpings until we arrived and went through the food line. Only then did they ask for additional servings.

It came as no surprise that the promising practice in which we were interested targeted Paisley students enrolled in the building trades class. Those students, while learning the craft, constructed the building used to house the course. It happened in Paisley, Oregon.

Of the many funded projects, we visited only those which met the selection criteria. They were considered successful because they had met their goals and because a person or a document was available to recreate the situation.

Understandably, the prevalence of excellence and innovation was exhilarating. Reading these creative ideas and then seeing them exceed expectations gave a whole new meaning to "education." We, Ralph and I, were convinced that this was the system in which we wanted to participate. We then started seeking opportunities in Oregon where our teaching backgrounds and experiences might make us attractive candidates.

Getting or changing jobs in 1976 was frustrating and difficult. Following the decrease in home construction and the bottom falling out of the lumber industry, Oregon school budgets were equally precarious. We were forced to redefine our area of job-hunting to "West of the Mississippi." Further, we agreed that whoever received a contract offer in his/her area of expertise would be the serious contender. Both of us had tenure in New York state jobs—jobs which paid very well. When no offers had been received by the end of August, we put our tails between our legs and flew back to Alfred, New York where we had the security of tenure.

During the few days before classes began, we stayed at Alfred's only motel. One day I arranged for an apartment, utilities, and ordered a vehicle. When I returned to the motel, Ralph was on the phone. He turned to me and asked, "Do you want to go to Pueblo, Colorado?" We had already talked about it and had this standing agreement about whoever got an offer . . . . I nodded in agreement and answered, "Yes." In the short version, this is how we came to move to Pueblo, Colorado.

The problem of getting to Pueblo was a bit complicated. When the call offering the position in Pueblo came through to New York in the late afternoon, I had just about enough time to get refunds on deposits for rental, etc. We contacted the car dealer and asked if he could have it ready for pick-up the following morning. Ralph decided he would ask for another year's leave without pay. If this were not granted, he had in hand a letter resigning—that meant, no more tenure.

Knowing the President's schedule, the following morning Ralph was able to accost him with his leave request. As the President started to go on his way after denying the leave request, Ralph handed him the resignation. Then Ralph joined me to drive the rental car 25 miles to Hornell where we took possession of the new car from the dealer.

After taking possession of the new car, we had to back-track with both cars to return the rental car to the Rochester airport. Finally, we were officially on our way driving west with the new car through the hot, dry, drought-parched country. We knew how much more comfortable air conditioning was from our experience in Muncie. To install air conditioning now would take too much time because we were on a tight schedule. Classes in Pueblo had already commenced.

Once we were in Kansas, we drove interminably on flat, dusty land. Ralph declared he would never drive across Kansas again. And, in the almost 30 years since that journey, he never has.

Each night, when we stopped traveling, we had called ahead to make reservations at our next destination. We did this consistently until the last stop was Pueblo. Thinking that Labor Day weekend would not be as heavily traveled, we came tootling along into Pueblo surprised to find that the inns were crowded. This was Friday, just preceding the big Labor Day weekend of the State Fair. We were lucky to be offered one of the two remaining available Holiday Inn rooms; but that room was only good for 3-4 days. The next day we located the campus and various other areas of the city.

Sunday we found a suitable apartment not too far from the college. Monday we caught our breath and Tuesday, Ralph "hit the bricks." He assumed his office as Head of the English Department at the then University of Southern Colorado (now University of Southern Colorado at Pueblo) and began a long history of teaching overloads. But teaching is the pursuit he loves.

To move into the apartment from the Holiday Inn was not time consuming. The only luggage we had was what we had carried on the plane. This consisted of one, lightly-packed suitcase per person—just enough for two or three days; the electric typewriter and 25 pounds of 100% rag paper necessary for typing Ralph's thesis.

As soon as A-1 Rental opened after the Labor Day holidays, our essential furniture was delivered. From A-l Rental Furniture I had rented two folding cots, two chairs, a card table and a black-and-white TV. We now had facilities for eating, sleeping, dressing and bathing. Somehow I found enough furnishings that we were able to move out of the Holiday Inn into our apartment in about three days.

Cleaning and making the apartment ready to receive our two partial loads of possessions (which were following us around the country) alternated with typing Ralph's "Magnum Opus." His draft of the document had been approved officially, so now the material had to be made ready for the printer.

Of course, we had contacted the storage firm in Corvallis, Oregon earlier, to send our furniture to Alfred, NY when his job in Alfred had been our destination. At this point, we had to re-contact Corvallis and ask them to divert the van to Pueblo. And New York furniture was released to come to Pueblo. The Oregon furniture was already on its way when we tried to re-direct it, but it was caught in Minnesota and successfully rerouted.

In about a week, our furniture from New York arrived. I chatted with the crew from the van until the driver finally said, "Until I have a bank check for the moving expense, we don't unload." So I hied myself to the nearest bank and returned with check in hand. I had just disposed of empty boxes and cartons the next day when the rest of the furniture arrived. This time I didn't have to be reminded of the payment arrangement. All I had to know was the name and the amount to cover the moving cost. At last we were moved, had our treasures around us and could catch our breath.

Now that we were moved and the completed manuscript of Ralph's Magnum Opus was at the printers, I had to face the fact I had a medical problem. For the past year, the doctor at Oregon State had advised that I had a tumor (which the doctor felt was benign) that might require a hysterectomy. He had nagged me at each visit and I had promised him and myself that once we were settled, I would pursue the matter.

Yes, exploratory surgery indicated the hysterectomy was necessary. It was performed without fuss, feathers, or complications. Not more than ten days later I started a part-time job in the English Department writing lab. This terminated at the end of the semester when a full-time instructor was selected.

Teaching opportunities didn't appear at spring semester, so I signed on as a Kelly employee. Beginning and leaving jobs or work situations had always been at the high end of the dread list for me. But my first assignment was pleasant and I made long-term friendships with the staff. After that my antipathy about beginnings and endings ceased.

Intermittent Kelly assignments were not satisfying. I felt as if I had made a jump into oblivion. I had earned my stripes, put in the time and effort, jumped all the hoops and finished with respect from my teachers and peers. Continuing in the field of education seemed closed to me.

My teaching assignments were lean, few, and far between. Never even half time. The final indignity came when I was removed from teaching a course in Linguistics for no given reason after meeting with the class three times. I had the necessary credentials—a masters in Linguistics— and I had taught the class once before without complaint. I felt disenfranchised, but there was no recourse. In my disappointment I destroyed my reference materials, resumes, letters of reference, class notes, and transcripts. These activities didn't make me feel any better, but they certainly made more shelf space.

Although not a full-time teaching opportunity, teaching international students to prepare them for an American-college, academic experience brought a new challenge. The student body represented many countries. Class size varied from six to a maximum of ten individuals. For the first time, I experienced teaching with supplementary materials provided by use of computers. This organization had specially-designed curriculum materials in reading, grammar, composition, and vocabulary. The small class sizes were ideal and the related training materials were well designed. But I had no experience using computers.

My previous computer experience was limited to punching cards. I didn't even know how to turn the machines on. And when I signed on for the teaching schedule, I didn't understand that part of the assignment was supervising my class of students in the computer lab an hour a day.

Looking far more at ease than I felt, I ventured awkwardly into the lab room where most students were working at computer keyboards. I asked one of the students I knew to be more fluent, "How do I turn the machine on?" He barely smiled as he answered my question by showing me the keys and the sequence. As he offered to help me further, I couldn't help thinking to myself what a wonderful teacher he would make. He didn't laugh or make fun of me; he very seriously demonstrated what I had asked for and then generously offered more help should I need it. Later, I found more evidence that this was an unusually courteous student—a real gentleman who went out of his way to be helpful to those he knew and even those he didn't know.

The curriculum materials were superlative: the computer program introduced the idea, gave a thorough explanation at the appropriate level, and then gave a ten- or twenty-question test. If the student answered all the questions correctly, the machine played a little tune. When other students heard the tune, they cheered and clapped their hands to indicate their approval. Everyone joined in reinforcing the success.

These computer lab lessons were very successful. In class we had been working on a special verb form—the use of verbs "was" and "were" when the sentence began with "if." The next day in class, the students all aced the test. I was surprised at the ease with which the students had conquered what American students found difficult. None of my high school or graduate English courses had dealt with the "if" situation in conditions contrary to fact.

I remembered having encountered this same language-usage problem in high-school German class. It remains in my memory because the German-born teacher spent three, 60-minute periods attempting to explain it. When, after three hours, we students admitted we still didn't understand, she announced there was no more time and we had to go on. However, these international students, using the computer materials (after I introduced the concept in a one-hour class), not only understood but they could also use the premise in their writing. So my splendid explanation and teaching were not, after all, the means by which they had attained mastery. The mastery came as a result of supportive materials used with the computers.

Between school sessions Ralph and I usually made an annual trip back East to visit family. What was different about the 1985 trip, first, was that I went alone; second, while I was in New York visiting Linda, I took a bad fall and twisted the right knee. This is the leg which had undergone knee surgery and surgical repair of two broken bones. Walking became so painful that I had to cut my trip short, go directly home, and miss seeing my widowed mother in Michigan.

In time, with rest, the knee settled down. But then my back and shoulders developed continuous, severe pain. At first, my response had been, "Nobody's going to monkey with my back." But as time went on and the pain wore me down, I became more receptive to surgery. The surgeon admitted he wasn't quite sure what the problem was. He later explained that the nerves in the back of my neck were being compressed. He described how he carefully moved the nerves out of the way, cleaned out more space for them and put them back. Recovery was uneventful except that for six weeks I had to wear a Philadelphia collar to protect the area. Wearing the collar was necessary except when in the bath or shower. At that time, the collars were made out of a plaster-type compound and were not washable. When I asked Sister Nancy, the surgeon's nurse, how to clean the collar she replied, "Just use lots of talcum powder."

I realized, after surgery, that full-time employment required more strength and endurance than I could muster. Luckily, about the time I was getting restless for want of a regular, work schedule, I checked in for my annual, physical exam. My doctor had heard that I had experience in medical transcription and his office was looking for such a person. Thus started seven pleasant years doing work I enjoyed surrounded by interesting people. I could set my own hours— usually three hours in the morning. This gave me back my prized independence, stimulated my brain and kept me in the world of people.

As I look back, I can see that I was already beginning to experience breathing problems. They first appeared in singing—yes, I still took lessons and sang in the choir. Why not? I certainly had something to sing about. And I enjoyed it. After all, I was here! But having enough breath pressure to hit a note on pitch became less frequent and also more frustrating. But it took several years before I could acknowledge I was no longer able to sing—either for myself, certainly not in public. I still miss being able to lose myself in someone else's music to express a feeling far beyond the scope of normal speaking—not that I ever wanted to be in opera or on Broadway. But once I had been able to regain control of the diaphragm after polio, belting out a meaningful idea or "selling a song" gave me a special high.

Then I noticed daytime sleepiness. I'd nod off while sitting in a chair—all but fall off the chair. Many times I slept during my appointment at the hairdresser's. Even more scary, I fell asleep driving, but fortunately I awakened right away and had no accident. The increasing fatigue and sleepiness were noted by the leader of the post-polio support group I had been attending. She kept nagging me to get a sleep study—to find out why I was so tired and draggy (and began to look so poorly as she later confided). Finally I agreed and my doctor referred me to one of the local hospitals for the test.

A sleep study, to me, is like spending a night at a motel while having various parts of the body connected by electrical pads which convey electrical impulses to a machine. These impulses are run through a computer program which prints out reports of how the various body parts are working. In my case, the computer figured out how much time I spent in each stage of sleep, how long it took to fall asleep, how many sleep disturbances or interruptions, how long the interruptions lasted and other details the doctors could use for diagnosis. When the oxygen saturation registered below a certain point, the test was discontinued and supplemental oxygen delivered.

What recommendations came out of the sleep study? The pulmonologist recommended a tracheotomy and the use of supplemental oxygen at night. My reaction to the "trache" (tracheotomy) was negative. I pointed out that in 1952, I had had one so I had a basis for making my decision. My personal opinion now was that a trache was an open wound looking for an infection. Although I didn't admit it, I was afraid that the care and maintenance of a trache would threaten my independence because I could raise only one hand to the area. Changing and cleaning a trache tube would probably require two hands. Making decisions such as this must be done on an individual basis. I had my own experience, handicap and reasons for disagreeing with the recommendations.

As fortune would have it, shortly after receiving this untenable recommendation, Easter Seals sponsored a polio conference in a city not far from home. The workshop I attended on non-invasive breathing proved to be just what I was looking for. Dr. Barry Make of National Jewish Hospital described and illustrated the use of non-invasive ventilators which mimic the body's breathing pattern. Non-invasive ventilation was designed as one alternative to tracheotomies. Based on that presentation, I asked my general practitioner to refer me to Dr. Make for a second opinion. The request was answered so quickly it surprised me.

The contact with Dr. Make resulted in a three-day hospital stay during which a second sleep study was performed. Blood tests were made every two hours to test for the presence of adequate oxygen and for the build-up of carbon dioxide. The BiPap ventilator (which mimics an individual's breathing pattern) was deemed appropriate for me to use during sleep and one such machine was brought for me to try during an afternoon nap.

Using a face mask was unfamiliar but not frightening. Cynthia, realizing I was getting into unfamiliar territory, brought her cassette tape player and some tapes of music she knew I liked. With the ear phones on and the face mask in place, listening to the music I fell asleep almost immediately. And I slept uninterrupted for two hours. The nap produced wonderful, restful sleep. Later I described my first sleep with the ventilator as ". . . a cross between satin sheets and good chocolate."

When I left the hospital to go home, it was with the assurance that my provider would bring to my house and install a ventilator that evening. The equipment was duly installed and its use explained before I went to bed that night. Later I asked Ralph if the whooshing sound the ventilator made kept him awake. His answer was that the noise reassured him that I was breathing without lengthy interruptions.

For the past ten years, the ventilator has contributed to my health and well-being. Improvement in the quality and duration of sleep has lessened both fatigue and pain. This compact, 35-pound device travels readily and accompanies me on the plane. (I don't trust it to the luggage department for if it were lost or damaged, I would be in deep trouble.) Traveling in the early 1990s was easier because airplane seat room allowed space for stowing the device under the seat in front of me. When I carried my own luggage, the ventilator was my carry-on. My suitcase was checked through with the other luggage. Now, seats are arranged with so little room that the ventilator has to be stowed in the overhead compartment. This change requires that either my husband, companion or some willing helper heave my carry-on into the overhead storage bin. Hefty athletes have been very responsive about helping when I am by myself.

My philosophy is that whenever possible, one should give to or help others in return for the many kindnesses, gifts and favors received. I think of it as saying "thank you" to others in need as an expression of my gratitude to those who helped me. In doing so I am expressing gratitude to individuals that I never saw and many others whose names or faces I never knew. And, it makes me feel good.

In addition to travel and working part time, I renewed interest in sewing. Friends invited me to join their quilt club. I discovered that piecing simple patterns was not too difficult with the machine. Hand sewing required more strength and dexterity than this right-handed person retained. However, when it came to quilting, I couldn't roll up and handle the standard-sized quilts with the batting and all. And I am too independent to ask someone else to do all that rolling to get the quilt mass under the machine's stitching foot. The alternative? A comforter. So, I made and tied several comforters. But the next generation much prefers blankets or down-filled comforters. This meant that I had no ready market for comforters. Well, that didn't work.

Recently I found a wonderful sewing teacher who offered classes for people like me who have difficulty finding clothing that fits. Polio survivors are only some of the people who don't fit off-the-rack garments or pattern sizes. Because I have a dropped right shoulder (from lack of shoulder girdle muscles) and because I have a flat rear, store-bought clothes seldom fit. Nor did I have the savvy to adapt patterns. But this teacher knew how to fit patterns. She taught us to sew for fun and success. She showed us how to make a sample "muslin" first. When the sample was fitted, we could then make the garment out of "fashion" fabric being sure that it would fit! That method had satisfaction guaranteed. In the process, I coined a short personal description: "I'm a classy lassie with an asymmetric chassis."

Another recent change came as a result of renewed interest in ham radio. In 1986 I found out that my favorite cousin, who had retired in California, had taken up radio and had received his ham (amateur) license. When he found out that I had used Morse code in the Navy, he suggested I take the amateur radio exam.

The day my license arrived, my husband and my teacher were installing the antenna for my "experienced" transceiver radio. I was so excited to communicate with London and Texas the first day. My cousin (call sign KA6NDX) and I (call sign N0LJP) chatted in Morse code over a period of several years. He had a far more powerful radio and antenna system on which I once reached Japan from his radio "shack"—the second bedroom of his home. From my shack, I exchanged signals with Canada, Texas, Illinois, New Jersey, Florida and a special one from the Queen Mary 2. Now that my cousin, KA6NDX, is a "dead key'—no longer with us—much of the joy and excitement have been lost too. But my vanity license plate reads N0LJP. If you are a ham radio operator and notice my call sign as you drive by, honk your horn.

Eating also underwent a fairly recent lifestyle change. Even though the right elbow and hand never did raise very high after acute polio, until about ten years ago I was able to handle eating irons with the right hand. But when food kept slipping off the fork, the soup spoon turned over and spilt the liquid, or the utensil just fell out of my fingers, I was grateful to be able to switch to the left hand. The change-over was not without frustration, but it was doable.

After I was smart enough to switch to the left hand, I found that I was able to wash my face, comb my hair, brush my teeth, eat and put on makeup with the left. These seldom considered as essential to activities of daily life are necessary to personal dignity and independence. I'm often reminded of a young priest in the area of Appalachia where we lived. When in dire need and resources were unavailable to him, he would say, "Wealth is having an alternative."

However, losing the ability to sing represented the loss of a vital part. For thirty years after acute polio, from singing I had drawn renewal, greater understanding—all those adjuncts which strengthen faith. Through music and song, words had additional layers of meaning which resonated deep in my gut.

After seven years of commuting 35 miles to a post-polio support group, I started a group here in Pueblo. I figured that although Pueblo is 100 miles north of the New Mexico state line, this also includes the southern part of the state. Pueblo, then, was the nearest place for a lot of polio survivors who weren't able to attend groups in the northern two-thirds of the state. Through this newer group, we offer friendship and share information which is becoming available through conferences and the internet.

The monthly, eight-page post-polio Newsletter I've written for the past nine years reaches about 200 individuals—some are survivors, others are caregivers or interested professionals. Although our local support meeting group is not sizable, members come when they are able to or when they want to exchange information. Polio survivors from as far as 100 miles distant are attending our meetings. Most of them depend on the Newsletter to keep abreast of developments in the field of post-polio survivorship. Probably the Newsletter is the most significant of my "give back" efforts. This is a way for me to say thanks to those who have given of their time, efforts and resources—people I have never met and never had a chance to express my gratitude to.

Were it not for encountering polio, probably none of my accomplishments would be worth writing about. To begin with, meeting my mortality head-on made me evaluate my life. Until that time I had never acknowledged that my two children were my most precious gifts. Living to see them grow to maturity became my driving force. To sing and to acquire the doctoral degree were two other, but subservient, goals. Looking back now, love was the incentive which made the other two goals possible.

The Great Spirit, that power beyond our own, who granted my requests also crossed my path with a wonderful helpmate. He is the man I am in love with and married to, the person I most admire both personally and professionally. It is he who smoothed the way and made many dreams possible for me and my children. This wonderful person married me forty years ago when I still managed as a passer—an able-bodied person. Now, although he seems to anticipate my new limitations even before I do, his love and support are always there to help me transit some of these rocky paths. He is ever "a soft place to fall."

Never have I seen anyone I would trade places with. I haven't been tempted to cry, "Why me?" Mine has been a wonderful, sometimes scary, often miraculous life. I am grateful for the challenges I encountered and the wonderful people I've been privileged to have met. Most of all, I am thankful that all my wishes were granted—especially that I have been permitted to see my daughters grow into beautiful, bright, charming individuals who are concerned stewards of the earth.

"Life is not a journey to the grave with the intention of arriving safely in a pretty and well-preserved body, but rather to skid in broadside, thoroughly used up, totally worn out, and loudly proclaiming, 'WOW! What a ride!'"

—————Author Unknown

About the Author

In 1969, the writer's husband declared that anyone who took 29 years to achieve a bachelor's degree ought to have something more than a piece of paper; so he had the parchment reproduced on a metal-and-wood plaque. Three more plaques followed: a master of science in English (1970), a master of arts in linguistics (1974), and an doctor of education in vocational business (1976) where the thesis researched and identified communication skills necessary for job-entry-level mechanics. Much of this academic preparation and writing occurred while teaching full time.

The writer authored Promising Practices published by Oregon State University. As a volunteer at the Cooperative Care Center (a local, crisis center), she wrote several successful grants. She also writes a monthly newsletter for the Pueblo and Colorado Springs, Colorado, Post-Polio Support Groups.

Printed in the United States
94949LV00003B/301-306/A